Cooking

with

Green

Tea

Avery

A MEMBER OF
PENGUIN PUTNAM INC.

Cooking with Green Tea

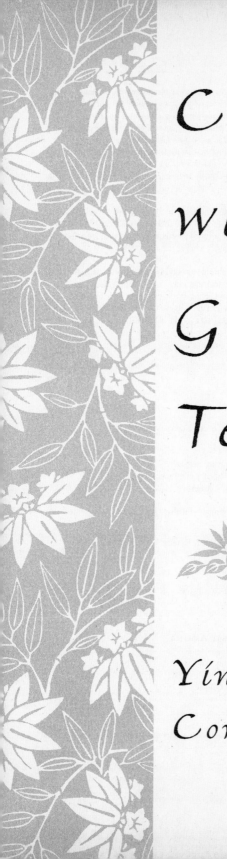

Ying Chang
Compestine

Most Avery books are available at special quantity discounts for bulk purchase for sales promotions, premiums, fund-raising, and educational needs. Special books or book excerpts also can be created to fit specific needs. For details, write Putnam Special Markets, 375 Hudson Street, New York, NY 10014.

Avery
a member of
Penguin Putnam Inc.
375 Hudson Street
New York, NY 10014
www.penguinputnam.com

Library of Congress Cataloging-in-Publication Data

Compestine, Ying Chang.
    Cooking with green tea/Ying Chang Compestine.
      p.   cm.
    Includes index.
    ISBN 1-58333-065-8
    1. Cookery (Tea).   2. Green tea.   I. Title.
TX817.T3C65   2000   00-28342
641.6'372—dc21

Printed in the United States of America

10 9 8 7 6 5 4 3 2 1

Book design by Jennifer Ann Daddio
Photography by Victor Giordano
Food styling by BC Giordano

Photograph of the author © Cooking Light magazine

To My Son and Sunshine,

Vinson (Ming Da) Compestine.

Every day you add so much joy

and happiness to my life!

ACKNOWLEDGMENTS

I have had the good fortune to receive support, friendship, professional guidance, care and love from many people.

I am very grateful to Martin Yan for his professional guidance and friendship. We both share a deep love of China. Martin, you are the master of fine Asian cooking.

I also want to thank John Duff at Penguin Putnam for his confidence and trust in my ability to write this series, and for his patience and professional guidance.

Throughout the years, I am blessed to receive the consistent support, guidance and friendship from the staff of *Cooking Light*. I am especially grateful to Doug Crichton, Rod Davis and especially Jill Melton.

Many thanks to the following people and companies: Tamara Parker at Calphalon, Kathleen McDonnell at Henckels, Mike Gilliland and Peter Williams at Wild Oats, Amelia Barrett at the Lauren Peck Agency, and Jeff Hamano at Zojirushi American Corporation.

A special thanks to my editor, Jeanette Egan, for her patience and professionalism, and her generous efforts in working with me to make it a great book.

I also want to extend my thanks to the following friends who cook, taste and critique my recipes. Their friendship brings a warm light to my life. Thank you, Diane and Fred Glover, Valerie and Dan Crecco, Lisa Rattenni, Susan Rampson, Amy Gahran, and Tom Vilot.

And last but not least, to my husband Greg, who tastes, critiques, and cheerfully does the dishes: Thank you for always encouraging me to pursue my dreams.

Contents

Cooking with Green Tea

"Not for all the tea in China . . ."

This common expression describes a big amount of trade-off for something extremely valuable. I wonder if the person who coined it had any idea just how right he was. In China, tea is more than a beverage. It is an intricate part of our culture: we use it to quench our thirst, as an ingredient in cooking, to toast friendship, as an offering to deities and ancestors, and yes, even as a medicine.

Over the years, I have promoted the health benefits of drinking tea to my friends and on my television show, *Yan Can Cook*. I have tried my hand at many dishes that included tea as an ingredient: Tea-Smoked Chicken and Shrimp Sautéed with Dragonwell Tea are two of my all-time favorites.

I met Ying many years ago and immediately was struck by her great energy, her boundless enthusiasm and her vast knowledge of teas. We share a great love for our native country, China, and on countless occasions

Ying was kind enough to enlighten me on many aspects of contemporary life in the mainland. An educator and a natural-born teacher, Ying has such an easy way of guiding her audiences to make their own discoveries on any subject.

I remember the many discussions we have had over the years on the topic of cooking with tea, and how I had lamented to her that there are so few good books on the subject. Well, I see that she has taken my comment to heart. *Cooking with Green Tea* is well written, colorful, and filled with delicious and easy-to-follow recipes that are right for every kitchen. They are certainly right for mine, and I wouldn't trade them for anything . . . not even for all the tea in China.

Chef Martin Yan
Yan Can Cook

Cooking with Green Tea

Just as Americans grow up drinking a variety of fruit juices, I grew up drinking a variety of teas. I also ate many dishes prepared with tea. Yes, "ate." In China green tea has been used in cooking almost as long as the Chinese have been drinking it. Tea has been popular in China since the Tang Dynasty (618–906 A.D.). For centuries we have revered it as a natural healer for body and soul.

One cup of regular green tea contains only about one-third the caffeine in a cup of coffee. Decaffeinated tea contains as many antioxidants as regular tea.

Health Benefits of Green Tea

Recently, researchers have found that green tea is a natural source of antioxidants and that it has the following health benefits:

Prevents cancer and heart disease

Restricts the increase of blood cholesterol

Controls high blood pressure

Lowers blood sugar levels

Controls inflammation

Suppresses aging

Refreshes the body

Fights viruses

Promotes weight loss

The antioxidants in green tea may have important health benefits. Antioxidants prevent or delay damage to your body's cells and tissues. They reduce the risk of heart attacks and protect the blood vessels that feed the heart and brain.

Hot and chilled green teas contain the same amount of antioxidant, but not the bottled ones. A study funded by the USDA found that bottled teas lack the major antioxidants, and some are loaded with sugar.

Researchers at the University of Kansas attributed green tea with 100 times the antioxidant strength of vitamin C, and 25 times that of vitamin E. A USDA study found that the antioxidant capacity of green tea is better than that of twenty-two various fruits and vegetables. A study conducted by the USDA Human Nutrition Research Center on Aging found that one cup of tea brewed for 3 to 5 minutes contains about the same amount of antioxidants as one serving of vegetables.

Researchers at Case Western Reserve University found that green tea may prevent inflammation from injury or from diseases such as arthritis. The antioxidants in green tea inhibit the Cox-2 enzyme, which causes inflammation.

Green tea may prevent skin cancer. Research at the University Hospital of Cleveland found skin damage from ultraviolet light was lower when the skin was protected by green tea. Studies from China and Japan indicate that green tea may also help prevent oral cancers.

Purdue University researchers found that green tea leaves are rich in EGCG, a compound that inhibits an enzyme required for cancer cell growth and that can kill cultured cancer cells with no ill effect on healthy cells.

According to Dr. Lester A. Mitscher, chair of the medical chemistry department at Kansas University and the author of *The Green Tea Book*, "The polyphenols—antioxidants found in green tea—have been found to be among the most effective antioxidants, more powerful than vitamins C and E." Dr. Mitscher recommends that people consume the equivalent of at least four cups of green tea per day, which contain 300 to 400 milligrams of polyphenols to maximize its health benefits.

Green Tea in Cooking

With the fast pace of life today, I find it hard to make the time for four cups of green tea every day. The Chinese solution is to incorporate green tea into cooking. You too can enjoy not only its unique flavor in your cooking, but a healthier mind and body.

This book introduces the different kinds of tea, along with step-by-step guidelines on how to brew and cook with green tea. Seventy imaginative recipes, all flavored with tea, are divided into chapters by their featured ingredients. You will find these delicious dishes easy to cook, and most of the ingredients and seasonings do not require a special trip to an Asian market. The majority of the recipes can be made with a nonstick wok or cooking pan.

As a bonus, based on the research indicating that green tea slows the absorption of carbohydrates and stimulates fat burning, I have developed a three-day cleansing and diet program. It will help you feel refreshed and energized and also lose 5 to 7 pounds.

It is my hope that this book presents another lesser known way of enjoying the flavor and health benefits of green tea—that of using it in cooking. If in addition to drinking green tea you start adding it to your own dishes, I will have met my goal.

About Tea

All teas come from the *Camellia sinensis* plant. Newly plucked leaves, considered "natural" or "fresh," are the source of the dried tea. The quality of a tea depends on the quality and condition of the fresh leaves. The younger the leaves of the plant, the higher their quality. The processing of tea, by inducing physical or chemical changes in the leaf, produces the three major types of tea:

+ Black tea is made from fully fermented leaves.
+ Oolong or red tea is partially fermented, and its flavor and color fall between those of black tea and green tea.
+ Green tea is made from unfermented leaves. Of the loose green teas, Gunpowder and Dragonwell are my favorites. Each leaf of Gunpowder is rolled into a pellet, which unfurls when the tea is brewed. It makes a dark green tea with a strong, pleasant flavor and long-lasting

aftertaste. Dragonwell makes a light green, fresh, mellow tea with a flowery aroma. When the best grade of Dragonwell is brewed, the leaves open up to reveal intact buds.

In addition to the main types of tea there are other kinds. Flavored teas are made by the addition of other plant leaves, flowers, roots, fruit or spices to the tea leaves. Herbal teas are made of other plant leaves, flowers, roots or spices but do not contain real tea.

Brewing Tea

Never boil water for tea in an aluminum teakettle or steep tea in plastic or aluminum. I like to use stainless teakettles, such as those with the porcelain enamel finish on steel made by Le Creuset. Stainless steel is nonreactive and does not absorb flavor or odors, thus providing the purest water for tea. The Le Creuset teakettles range from $40 to $70 in price.

I prefer to brew tea in Yixing teapots, which have been used in China since the Sung Dynasty (960–1279). These pots are made of purple clay enriched with natural minerals. The pot develops a rich patina and "seasoning" with use that enhances the taste and aroma to bring out the best of a fine tea.

Other good choices for teapots are china, porcelain or stainless steel. Always fill your teacup or teapot with hot water to preheat it and discard the water before adding the tea and the brewing water. Covering the teapot or cup helps the tea leaves unfurl, which also helps loose tea leaves settle to the bottom.

Fresh bottled spring water is the best choice for making tea. The second choice would be filtered water. Tap water contains chemicals that can alter the taste of a brew. Different types of tea require different temperatures of water.

GREEN TEAS AND LIGHT FLOWERY HERBALS

For the best flavor and the most infusions, brew green tea with 160–170F (71–76C) water. This is when the water first begins to stir. It's restless but not simmering. It is better to steep green tea at a lower temperature for a little longer than to force the leaves to give up their essence with high temperatures, which will end up making a bitter brew. According to research, after 3 to 4 minutes of brewing time, you will get all the health benefits from the green tea.

OOLONG, SEMIFERMENTED AND BLACK TEAS

These teas do best with near-boiling water, about 195F (91C). This is when the water is dancing and hissing. There are bubbles rising across the entire surface; it's starting to steam, on the verge of boiling.

HEAVY BLACK TEAS AND HERBAL TEAS WITH ROASTED INGREDIENTS

Water at a full, rolling boil is needed to release the full flavors of heavy traditional black tea, such as Chinese puerh teas and hearty herb blends.

Using Tea Bags

According to the American Tea Council, tea is regularly consumed by more than half the population in the United States. Eighty percent of tea is made using tea bags, while the rest of it is brewed from loose tea. After I came to America, I found myself using tea bags instead of loose tea. Some dedicated tea drinkers insist that loose leaf renders the finest flavor and aroma. Most of us would be hard pressed to tell a difference in taste.

According to research, the finer the green tea, the more health benefits you get. Since the tea in a bag is finely chopped, you may get more benefits by using tea bags.

In this book, I brewed from tea bags for soup bases, marinades and sauces. To get the most of green tea's delicate flavor and health benefits, in these recipes I use two to three times as much tea as I do to make tea for drinking. Use pure green tea for cooking soups, main dishes and vegetables. Fruit-flavored and jasmine green teas can be used for desserts, sauces, smoothies and drinks.

To use the tea from tea bags for seasoning: Cut open the tea bags and remove the contents, discarding the empty bags. Heat a wok or frying pan with oil. Add the tea and cook until the tea releases its flavor before adding the rest of the ingredients.

When a recipe calls for loose tea, you can also substitute the tea from tea bags in most instances. Because the tea in tea bags is finer than loose tea, there are some recipes where only loose tea will work. Two tea bags contain about ½ tablespoon loose tea.

BREWING TEA BAGS FOR COOKING

Add a little steaming water to the teapot or cup and swirl the water to warm the teapot. Discard the water.

Place 2 to 4 tea bags in the pot. Immediately pour 1¼ cups boiling water over the tea bags. Cover and infuse for 2 to 3 minutes. Discard the tea bags. This makes 1 cup of very strong tea. Even when the recipe calls for less than 1 cup, I still make the larger amount. Use this liquid according to the recipes.

SMOKING WITH TEA

Cut open the tea bags and mix the tea with the other smoking ingredients. Discard the bags. You can also use loose tea.

Using Loose Tea

BREWING TEA LEAVES FOR COOKING

The Chinese have been cooking with high-quality green tea leaves for centuries. We use dry leaves as a seasoning, the brew as a sauce base, and the infused leaves as vegetables. I have found that the best teas for using as a vegetable or a seasoning are Dragonwell (Longjing) or Gunpowder. Any high-quality green tea is good for brewing tea for a soup base. I prefer to use pure green tea for everything except some sauces, desserts, smoothies and drinks—with them I prefer to use a flavored tea such as lemon. Lemon-flavored green tea is also good for seafood and some meat dishes. Experiment with different teas and find your favorite combinations.

When using dry tea leaves as a seasoning, add them to the heated oil like any other seasoning.

When cooking with tea leaves, first brew or steam the leaves. When brewing you need the leaves fully infused, so don't use a tea ball or infusing basket. Infuse loose green tea for 5 minutes. Try to think of the tea leaves as delicate leafy vegetables. Another way to infuse tea leaves is to steam them until infused before adding to the dish.

INFUSING TEA LEAVES TO USE
AS A VEGETABLE

Warm the teapot or cup by swirling steaming water in it. Discard the water. Place 1 teaspoon loose tea into the pot. Immediately pour ½ cup boiling water over the tea. Cover and let the leaves infuse for about 5 minutes, or until the leaves unfurl. This will make 1 tablespoon infused leaves. Save the liquid for a sauce and use the leaves for cooking.

STIR-FRYING TEA LEAVES

Heat oil in a nonstick wok or cooking pan over medium-high heat and add tea leaves. Cook until fragrant, just a few seconds. If using Gunpowder tea, you will see the little balls unfurl as they release a wonderful fragrance.

STEAMING TEA LEAVES TO USE AS A VEGETABLE

Place 1 teaspoon loose tea leaves in a vegetable steamer. Steam over medium-high heat for 10 minutes, until leaves soften. This will make ½ tablespoon infused tea leaves. Use the leaves according to the recipes.

USES FOR TEA

THE CHINESE USE TEA AS MEDICINE, IN BEAUTY PRODUCTS AND FOR OTHER PURPOSES. DO NOT DISCARD CONTENTS OF TEA BAGS, TEA LIQUID AND TEA LEAVES LEFT OVER FROM COOKING OR BREWING, BECAUSE THEY CAN BE USED FOR MANY OF THE PURPOSES LISTED HERE. THE LIQUID TEA BREWED FOR COOKING IS STRONGER THAN THAT USED FOR DRINKING, BUT IT CAN BE DILUTED WITH HOT WATER AND USED AS A BEVERAGE.

HEALTH AND BEAUTY

+ SOAK A TOWEL IN COLD TEA; PLACE THE TOWEL ON SUN-BURNED SKIN TO HELP COOLING AND HEALING.
+ USE TEA TO EASE SWELLING AND ITCHING.
+ USE STRONG TEA AS DISINFECTANT ON LACERATIONS OF THE SKIN.

- Press rehydrated tea leaves on an affected tooth to stop pain and swelling.
- Use strong tea to treat fungal foot infections, bathing the foot twice a day for 10 minutes for several weeks.
- Chewing rehydrated tea leaves cleanses the breath. Rinse the mouth with strong tea for cleaning.
- Soak a towel in warm tea, and place the towel on tired eyes to refresh them.
- Stuff a small pillow with dried, used tea leaves. It is believed that the tea-stuffed pillow ensures good sleep, promotes clear thinking and improves your mood.
- Wash the face with warm tea to treat pimples and skin rashes.
- Rinse freshly washed hair with strong tea for shine and softness.
- Bathing in mint-flavored green tea will rejuvenate the skin and have a cooling effect.

OTHER USES

- Spread tea around the roots of garden plants, especially roses and peppers. With used tea bags, tear open the bag and use the tea. Because used tea leaves contain organic matter, they make a good fertilizer for plants.
- Add used tea leaves to your compost pile.
- Burn dry tea leaves in a pot to drive mosquitoes away.

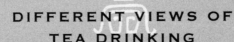

DIFFERENT VIEWS OF
TEA DRINKING

HISTORIANS BELIEVE THAT BUDDHIST MONKS INTRODUCED TEA TO JAPAN BETWEEN THE TANG (618) AND SUNG (1279) DYNASTIES.

JAPAN ADOPTED ITS OWN FASHION OF TEA DRINKING. THERE, TEA DRINKING IS A STYLIZED RITUAL DESIGNED TO CREATE A SENSE OF SPIRITUAL PEACE, SERENITY AND HARMONY WITH NATURE. MORE FOCUS IS GIVEN TO THE STEPS OF TEA PREPARATION THAN TO THE DRINKING OF THE TEA.

IN CHINA, TEA IS DRUNK MORE FOR ENJOYMENT AND IS A PART OF DAILY LIFE.

Cooking Basics

In this chapter you will find all the information you need to successfully prepare the recipes in the book, from the special equipment that will make cooking easier to helpful techniques to a list of the ingredients used throughout. Even if most of the ingredients and techniques are familiar to you, reading this chapter before starting the recipes will help you learn new skills and sharpen old ones.

Tools

KNIVES

No tool is more important in the kitchen than a good-quality knife. It will save you time and make cooking more enjoyable. Ten years ago, I received a pair of Henckels knives as a wedding gift. Since then I have been adding Henckels knives to my knife collection. The latest Henckels Twinstar Plus knives stay sharp for years. You may never need to resharpen them.

The key is to find a pair of knives that fit your hand and feel comfortable to use day after day. I find that large and heavy knives are too much to handle. My 8-inch chef's knife is the one I use the most.

RICE COOKER

I use my rice cooker more often than any other kitchen appliance. It stays on my kitchen counter all the time. Zojirushi makes a variety of sizes and styles of rice cookers. They range from a basic one costing $30 to an upscale one costing about $100, with a warmer feature that will keep your rice warm for up to 12 hours.

STOVETOP GRILLING PAN

This is a frying pan with parallel ridges on the bottom. It comes in round and square shapes. I fell in love with indoor grilling after I got a round Calphalon grilling pan. Since less of the food's surface comes in contact with the pan and its nonstick surface, you need less oil. I use a grilling pan to make our family's favorite dish, Spicy Green Tea Grilled Broccoli (page 131). The ridges sear the food and simulate grill marks while the flavorful juices remain in the pan, keeping the food moist and tender. Grilled food requires less seasoning. Even better, I can grill all year round, even when a big snowstorm hits Colorado. A lid and a kitchen fan help reduce smoke to a minimum. (The lid for my 12-inch wok fits my grilling pan.)

WOK

Not long after our wedding, Greg and I went back to China. One of my old aunts came all the way from the countryside to bring us a special wedding gift, a wok and a spatula. Her advice to me about marriage? "A couple is like a wok and a spatula, sometimes they make a lot of noise but in the end you get to enjoy a wonderful meal." In China, it is common for a newly married couple to receive gifts with a double meaning. Unfortunately, the wok didn't fit in our suitcase, but the advice stayed with us.

To save time cleaning, and to cut down the amount of fat in your food, choose a nonstick wok or a chef's pan, which I find works just as well. It is a little smaller than a wok but the shapes are similar. Many times I have found myself using the Calphalon chef's pan for quick and simple meals. I also use the chef's pan to cook soup and boil noodles. The shape of the wok and the chef's pan not only conducts heat well, but the high sides let you freely stir ingredients without spilling the food.

Now many companies make nonstick products. It is worth buying a high-quality one, which will last a lifetime, rather than a low-quality one where the coating peels off in months. Since woks come in different sizes and weights, find one that fits your needs. If you cook for one or two persons, a small 10-inch wok or a 4-quart chef's pan may be sufficient. A large family may want a 14-inch or larger wok. Buy one that comes with a lid. I like to cover the wok when I first put in the food. It protects you from spattering oil and saves time cleaning the cooktop afterwards. If your wok comes with a steam rack, you can also use it as a simple steamer.

YIXING TEAPOTS

Yixing, just a few miles up China's famous Yangtze River, is the home of Chinese pottery. Yixing pottery is famous for its unique, elegant forms, elaborate craftsmanship, earthy colors and functional performance. Originating some time during the Northern Sung Dynasty (960–1279), Yixing pottery was developed over several hundred years from the Sung to the Yuan Dynasty and eventually matured in the early Ming Dynasty (1368). In the Ming Dynasty, Yixing teapots became a necessity in teahouses and were highly valued by the upper classes. They were considered luxuries for the high officials of court and royal households. Later they were spread to the common people and introduced to Europe and rest of the world.

They are made of purple clay enriched with natural minerals. The fired clay contains tiny air pockets, which provide insulation. Yixing teapots are made without an interior glaze so that with use, the pot develops a rich patina and "seasoning" that enhances the tea's color and taste and brings out the best of a fine tea. To enjoy the full aroma of tea, the Chinese always use the same type of tea in the same pot, that is, green tea for one pot, black tea in another. The residual flavors of the different types of tea should not cross over into each other. Do not clean the teapot with soaps or detergents, because they can be absorbed by the clay and affect the taste of the tea. After all, in ancient China, dish soap was not available. Clean the teapot by rinsing it with plain hot water only.

Yixing pots come in different shapes, sizes and prices. Because of their porous quality and incredible designs, these teapots have become collector's items. Some teapots with breathtaking designs are for collectors and don't function well for pouring tea. Prices range from $30 for machine-made pots to more than $1,000 for one hand-made by a ceramic artist. The teapots range in capacity from ½ cup up to 4 cups.

Look for a one with a traditional, classic design. Unless you are a collector, $40 to $80 will give you a beautiful, well-designed machine- or handmade pot. Look for one that can brew at least 2 cups of tea. Both the Celestial Seasonings and Water and Leaves tea companies carry Yixing teapots. For more selections, check out the Web site www.yixing.com.

Seasoning your Yixing teapot: Line the bottom of a deep cooking pot with a dish towel. Add a few inches of cold water. Place the teapot, without the lid, on top of the towel. Add sufficient water to cover the pot.

Bring the water to a boil. Reduce heat to medium-low. Let simmer for 30 minutes. This will purify the pot, releasing any wax left over from the manufacturing process. Let the pot cool in the water.

Remove the pot. Place 4 tea bags or 4 tablespoons of tea leaves in the pot. Fill the pot with boiling water. Cover and let it cool.

Discard the tea. Rinse the teapot with warm water. Now you are ready to enjoy your teapot.

Techniques

The following techniques are used throughout this book. Mastering these basic skills will make it easier to cook healthy quick meals.

CUTTING TECHNIQUES

When you slice and shred, the objective is to create pieces of uniform size that will cook evenly.

Slicing: Hold the food firmly on the cutting board with one hand while the other hand holds the knife firmly. Cut the food straight down into very thin slices.

Shredding: Cut the food into ⅛-inch slices, then stack several slices and cut them lengthwise into ⅛-inch-thick matchstick pieces.

Mincing: Shred the food, then dice the shreds. One hand firmly holds the knife handle while the other holds down the blunt edge of the knife blade. Rock the knife up and down to mince the food evenly. Seasoning ingredients and garnishes such as herbs should be minced. Mincing makes the ingredients small enough to release all of the flavor into the dish, or to give the dish a light touch of color.

GARNISHING

This is the final touch to ensure that your creation becomes a "masterpiece." Keep it simple. Even two sprigs of cilantro or a sprinkling of minced red bell pepper add an artistic finish to the dish.

MIXING SAUCES

Many recipes in this book call for a sauce to be added to the dish. Always prepare the sauce before you start cooking. Make sure the mixture is smooth and well blended before adding it to the dish. For dipping sauces, the longer the dry ingredients marinate, the stronger the flavor. Refrigerate sauces in a sealed container.

SIMMERING

This technique is used for soups, sauces and stews. Simmering is a slow-cooking process that helps the ingredients absorb more flavor from each other and the sauce. Immerse the food in just enough boiling water to cover it. Bring the water back to a boil and then reduce the temperature to below the boiling point.

SMOKING

Smoking uses aromatic ingredients like orange peel, rice or green tea to give food a robust aroma. Traditional smoking methods tend to smoke your whole kitchen along with the food. These methods also tend to damage your favorite pan.

Experimentation perfected this method: Line the bottom of a large, nonstick, stainless steel pot with foil. Place all the smoking ingredients on top of the foil. Place the food on a steam rack. Cover tightly with foil, sealing the edges around the pot, and cover with a lid to seal in the smoke. Place over medium-high heat and smoke as directed in the recipe. Don't turn on the heat until you have sealed and covered the pot. This way only the food will get the smoky flavors, not your kitchen.

When done, turn off the heat and take out the food. Quickly re-cover the pot and keep covered while it cools. Once cool, discard the foil and smoking ingredients, which will be stuck to the foil. Not much cleaning is required, and the bottom of your pot is not damaged. To be safe, always use an old pot, and don't use a pot with a nonstick surface.

STEAMING

Steaming is the second most widely used cooking method in China. Steamed food is cooked by suspending the food over boiling water. It is an excellent method of cooking low-fat yet delicious food.

When steaming food, always check the water level often, and replenish the water as necessary. The food must remain above the water level and not get wet. When lifting the lid during steaming, always lift it up away from you so your hand is not exposed to the scalding steam. If you don't have a Chinese bamboo steamer, you can still use the following utensils.

Using a wok as a steamer: You will need a metal vegetable steam rack and a lid. To prevent the metal rack from scratching the bottom of a nonstick wok or pan, set the rack on a heatproof plate. If you don't have any kind of rack, place a small heatproof bowl filled with water in a large wok or pot. Use this bowl to support a larger heatproof owl containing the food. If the top bowl is deep enough to prevent water from coming into contact with the food, the water in the pot can cover the supporting bowl. Make sure that the water won't get into the food as it boils.

Using a large pot as a steamer: I like a vegetable steam rack that fits snugly over the top of the pot. Pour several cups of water into the pot and bring to a boil. Stack one to three steam racks over the pot and cover with a lid. This way you can steam more than one dish at a time.

Scanpan USA makes a stainless steel steamer that allows you to stack up to three layers onto a 10¼-inch pot.

If you have a folding steam basket, place a heatproof bowl in the bottom of the pot so that the food in the basket remains above the water. Add about 2 inches of hot water to the pot. Place the steam basket on the bowl. Place the food in the basket or on a heatproof plate that will fit on the basket, and place it in the basket. Bring the water to a boil. Cover and steam as directed in the recipe. Replenish the water as needed.

Steaming leftover foods: Steaming is one of the best methods of reheating food. It warms food without cooking it further and adds some moisture. To reheat rice, noodles and braised dishes, bring the water to a simmer but do not boil. Steam the food over medium-low heat to prevent overcooking.

STIR-FRYING

Stir-frying is the most common Chinese cooking technique. It is also a good way to cook healthy and fast meals. With a nonstick wok or cooking pan you need very little oil. Most stir-fried dishes take only minutes to prepare. Because the cooking time is short, the food retains its natural flavors, nutrients and textures.

Stir-frying can be a little intimidating at first. The following steps will ensure your successful and safe stir-frying.

Prepare the ingredients correctly: To ensure even and fast cooking, most of these recipes call for thinly sliced or shredded ingredients. This is when you will appreciate a good set of knives. I use chopping as a form of meditation. Put on some classical music, and chop, chop, chop. If you don't have time or have your own form of meditation, don't let that stop you from stir-frying. You can always use precut meats, bagged salad and even frozen vegetables. That is what I do many weeknights.

Assemble all the ingredients: Stir-frying is like getting on a roller coaster—once you start, there's no stopping. So make sure you have everything cut, meats marinated and sauces mixed. Arrange everything near the wok, including the serving plate and garnishes.

Set the table: That's right! Stir-fry food tastes best when hot. You don't want your hot creation getting cold and soggy. (If dinner is delayed, place the food in a covered dish and keep it warm in an oven set on warm.)

Order of cooking: Stir-frying is usually done in batches, and the order in which ingredients are added is important. Aromatic seasonings like green tea, ginger and garlic usually go in first, followed by meats or seafood, and hard vegetables such as carrots go in before softer ones such as spinach and cabbage. Add in sauce when all the food is halfway cooked.

Begin to cook: Use high heat. Heat the wok or cooking pan for 30 seconds before adding the oil. Drizzle in the oil, usually no more than 2 tablespoons. Swirl it to coat the surface. Don't wait until the oil is too hot. If you can hold your hand above the wok and can feel the heat, it's ready. If the recipe calls for dry green tea leaves, garlic, ginger or chile pepper, this is the time to add it. With practice you can judge by the cooking sound and smell. The purpose here is to flavor the oil and release the fragrance of the seasonings.

Quickly add other ingredients and cover immediately to prevent splattering. Keep the food moving by giving the wok a couple of good shakes. After a couple of seconds of shaking, you are safe to open the lid and start stir-frying. Most of the water has cooked off.

Stir: Use your spatula to toss the food over the surface of the wok or pan, so that everything cooks evenly. I prefer to use one of the new heat-resistant silicone spatulas such as the Le Creuset ones, which can resist temperatures up to 650F (345C).

TASTING

Don't forget to taste the dish before you put it on the serving plate. Many recipes call for salt and pepper to taste. This is the time to adjust the seasoning. I always save sesame oil to the end, since its flavor tends to evaporate in high heat.

WATER-BLANCHING

This technique softens up vegetables and enhances their vibrant colors. It is commonly used for firmer vegetables such as broccoli and carrots. Place the vegetable in boiling water and boil until the color is brighter—several minutes. Drain and rinse under cold water to stop the cooking process. In most cases, blanching food precedes stir-frying, which is used to complete the cooking. The blanched vegetables can be added to soup, served with sauces or used as a garnish.

Ingredients

My pantry and refrigerator are my treasure boxes. I go to these boxes when I am happy and hungry, when I am social and creative. With the following "treasures" on hand, a healthy and delicious meal is just minutes away.

My home in Boulder is one hour away from the nearest Asian market districts. Yet thanks to an explosion of interest in healthy foods, and Asian foods in particular, I don't have to travel that far. I can now easily find my ingredients in the Asian sections of my local health food stores and supermarkets. You can even order many of the ingredients listed here from your home; check the resources section at the end of the book.

Staples (Dry Treasures)

Canola Oil: I prefer using canola oil to other types of cooking oil. Rich in monounsaturated fats and low in saturated fats, it also contains a good amount of linolenic acid, an essential omega-3 type fat. With its mild, bland taste it is an all-purpose cooking oil that doesn't interfere with flavors. You can substitute other vegetable oils for canola oil.

Chili Garlic Paste: Made from red or green chiles, garlic, salt and other seasonings, it is sold in jars. Look for varieties that are low in sodium. Refrigerate after opening.

Curry: This seasoning is available in powder and paste forms. Curry powder is a combination of ground spices, including cumin, coriander, turmeric, cinnamon and more. Curry pastes come in a range of flavors and degrees of spiciness. All of them contain spices and oil. Red curry contains red chilies; green curry contains green chiles. Yellow curry contains a blend of dried spices. Try them all and find the type that fits your taste. I prefer curry powder because I can better control the amount of oil and spices in the dish. Curry has a very strong flavor, so a little can make a big impression.

Fish Sauce: Made from fermented shrimp or fish, this thin, clear, brown sauce has a very fishy odor and salty taste. Don't let the smell stop you from trying it. The fishy smell greatly diminishes after cooking. It is popular throughout southeast Asia and southern China. I find that green tea mellows its smell and enhances its flavor. It is sold in bottles in the Asian section of supermarkets, health food stores and Asian specialty markets. It will keep for several months after opening without refrigeration.

Five-Spice Powder: Also known as five-flavored powder, this brownish powder is a mixture of star anise, Sichuan peppercorns, fennel, cloves and cinnamon. It has a pungent, fragrant, spicy and sweet taste. It has a long shelf life when kept in a tightly sealed jar.

Green Tea: Have loose and bagged green tea on hand. Green tea comes in many different types. Have several in your pantry. They come in handy when you want to give your food a certain flavor, and they go well with your dessert. Store the tea in a tightly sealed container. Glass and ceramic containers are the best choice. Store the tea in cool, dry and dark place.

Nori: A nutritious sea vegetable that is a good source of iron and iodine. It has an olive-brown color and comes in threads, sheets, strips and granules. Some varieties are dry and must be soaked in warm water and softened before using. Other varieties have been roasted and seasoned and require no presoaking. The recipes call for toasted nori (also called yaki nori). Store in a sealed container in your pantry for up to 6 months.

Miso: A fermented soy food made from soybeans and grains. There are many varieties on the market. Try to find a brand that is low in sodium and preservative-free.

NOODLES
The following noodles can be substituted for each other. To substitute fresh for dry noodles, add one-fourth more. Always soak dry

bean and rice noodles before cooking, except for wheat noodles. Use angel hair or linguine as a substitute for thin bean and rice noodles; use fettuccine as a substitute for wide rice noodles.

+ *Bean threads* are made from ground mung beans. They come in various lengths and thicknesses. These fine white noodles are sold in neat bundles in plastic packages. They will keep in a dry, tightly sealed container for up to 6 months. They are popular in soups, cold noodle dishes and fillings.
+ *Rice noodles* are made from long-grain rice flour. These white noodles come in a variety of shapes and thickness. Refrigerate fresh ones and cook within two days. Keep the dry form in a tightly sealed container in a dry and cool place for up to six months. Rice noodles are popular in stir-fry dishes, cold noodle dishes and soups.
+ *Wheat noodles* are made from wheat flour and water. Sometimes eggs are added. They are sold fresh or dry and come in various shapes.

RICE AND RICE PRODUCTS

+ *Glutinous rice*, also known as sweet or sticky rice, is a variety of short-grain rice with a short, round, pearl-like shape. High in starch, when cooked it turns translucent, soft and sticky. It is widely used in Asian festival dishes and desserts.
+ *Long-grain rice*, with long slender grains that are about four times as long as they are wide, is the favored rice in China. When cooked, the rice separates easily and is less starchy than short-grain. It is perfect for making fried rice dishes.
+ *Short-grain rice*, with round, plump oval grains, is preferred in the eastern areas of Asia. High in starch, the rice sticks together when cooked. It is used as an accompaniment to main dishes, in Japanese sushi and in Chinese congee.

- *Sweet rice flour* is made with glutinous rice. It is widely used in Asian desserts. It is not the same as rice flour made from long-grain rice. Asian and some health food stores carry it in small plastic packages.
- *Rice vinegar*, made from rice, has a less acidic taste than cider or wine vinegar. It comes in black and red. Black vinegar is dark in color and mild in flavor; red vinegar is sweet and spicy in taste. You can substitute cider vinegar for both.
- *Rice wine*, made with glutinous rice, yeast and spring water, has a rich, sweetish mellow taste. Dry sherry can be substituted, but not regular wines.
- *Rice wrappers* are thin, translucent sheets made with rice and water. They are the southeast Asian version of the tortilla, used for wrapping various fillings. Before using, briefly soak in warm water till soft. Store in a dry and cool place for up to 6 months.

Sesame Oil: Made from toasted sesame seeds, it has a strong nutty flavor and aroma. It is so flavorful that a small amount will add a distinctive taste to dishes. Since it heats rapidly and the flavor evaporates easily, add it to the dish at the end of cooking, or in a sauce, but do not use it as a cooking oil. It is sold in bottles and is best stored in a cool dark place. Don't refrigerate; it will turn cloudy.

Soy Sauce: Made from fermented soybeans, water, salt and sometimes wheat. The two main types are light and dark. Dark soy sauce is matured longer. It is thicker and tastes stronger than light soy sauce. It is used for flavor and for added color in dishes. The light sauce is used in dipping sauces. You can also find low-sodium brands on the market. I like to use naturally fermented soy sauce, which you can find at health food stores and in the Asian section of some supermarkets. To reduce sodium in regular soy sauce at home, simply replace half of the soy sauce called for in the recipe with lemon juice, rice wine or water. Soy sauce will keep for several months without refrigeration.

Teriyaki Sauce: Commercially available; made of soy sauce with additional ingredients such as pineapple juice, chile pepper, ginger, garlic or sugar added. It has a savory, sweet flavor and works well as a marinade. It is an ideal sauce for quick cooking, because you get several ingredients in one bottle. Refrigerate after opening. I prefer the Kim's brand, made with the natural ingredients.

Fresh Ingredients (Fresh Treasures)

Baby Bok Choy: Has dark green leaves and a thick white stem, 6 to 8 inches long. It is a smaller, young version of bok choy and tastes sweeter and is less fibrous.

Bamboo Shoots: These come from the tips of bamboo stalks. The crisp, pale flesh has a mild flavor. Rinse canned or bottled shoots in cold water before using. Look for shredded shoots to save time. If you are lucky enough to find fresh shoots, give them a try. Wash, peel and blanch the shoots in boiling water for 10 minutes before cooking.

Cilantro (Chinese parsley or fresh coriander): It has a uniquely fragrant, slightly musky flavor. It adds flavor to a variety of dishes.

Grape Leaves: The easy way to get fresh ones is from your own grape plant; use only leaves that have not been sprayed with chemicals. You can also find them frozen in many stores.

CHILE PEPPERS

There are a wide variety of fresh and dried chiles to choose from. You can choose and substitute among chiles based on your passion for spicy food. Choose fresh chiles without brown patches or black spots.

After handling chiles, wash your hands, knives and cutting board thoroughly with soapy water and rinse well. Don't touch your eyes, lips or other sensitive areas for several hours. You may want to wear rubber gloves when you prepare very hot chiles.

+ *Jalapeño* is a medium-hot chile. This cone-shaped chile is usually shiny green and turns red when ripe. It is the standard barometer for spiciness among chiles.
+ *Fresno* is a hot chile. This California-grown chile resembles the jalapeño but is slightly broader; about 2 inches long and 1 inch wide.
+ *Serrano* is a very hot chile. It is slender, about ½ inch long and much hotter than the jalapeño. It comes in green, red and yellow colors; it also comes dried.

Coconut Milk: Some Asian dishes call for coconut milk, which is high in fat, especially saturated fat. Reduced-fat coconut milk is also available, but it still is not a low-fat food. In this book I have substituted coconut-pineapple juice, coconut powder and soy milk.

Dumpling Skins (Gyoza): These round wrappers vary in thickness. Thicker ones are good for boiled dumplings and the thinner ones are better for pan-fried dumplings.

Garlic: This perennial plant produces round bulbs of familiar garlic cloves. Look for firm bulbs that aren't shriveled and have no broken skin. Elephant garlic is twice as large as regular garlic, is easier to peel and has a milder flavor.

Ginger Root: This knobby root has a shiny, smooth, golden skin and a yellow-green interior. It has a spicy, pungent flavor and tantalizing aroma. It is used to season many Asian dishes. Ginger root is available in the produce section of most supermarkets. Look for hard, heavy, unwrinkled fresh ginger root and store in a plastic bag in the refrigerator. Stale ginger starts to turn blue from oxidation. Fresh ginger skin doesn't need to be peeled. Dried and stem ginger should not be substituted for fresh ginger.

Green Soybeans (Edamame): These green legumes have a very mild taste and are packed with nutrition. When I discovered frozen green soybeans in my health food store, I filled my freezer with them. Some grocery stores and many Asian markets also sell soybeans. You can even buy them fresh at some farmer's markets. Eat only the beans and discard the pods. Frozen green soybeans that have already been removed from the pods are available at some health food stores and Asian markets.

Leeks: A member of the onion family; has long white bulbs and long-bladed soft green leaves. It has a sweeter and less pungent taste than regular onions. Leeks are often very muddy or sandy, so it is important to clean them well. The easiest way to clean leeks is to first slice off and discard the root end and tough outer green leaves. Then split the bulb lengthwise, separating the layers of the bulb and leaves. Soak them in cold water for 5 minutes, then gently remove the stubborn grit under running water with a brush.

Lemon Grass: This herb has a delicate lemon aroma and flavor. Fresh lemon grass is a green 3-foot-long stalk. Use only the 5-to-7-inch bulblike base. Peel and discard the external tough, dry leaves. Shredded bulbs are used to flavor soup while minced bulbs are used in sauces. Use lemon peel as a substitute. You can find lemon grass in the produce department of some supermarkets.

MUSHROOMS

Mushrooms are an easy way to add flavor to your cooking. Their delicate flavors go well with green tea. Thanks to the extraordinary variety of foods available today, we can now find a variety of fresh mushrooms in stores. If you can't find the kind called for in a recipe, feel free to substitute one for another. Most mushrooms are available in plastic packages or in bulk. For fresh mushrooms, look for firm, dry flesh free of blemishes. Buy mushrooms as you need them because they do not store well.

- *Enoki* is a cream-colored, long-stemmed, small-capped mushroom with a delicate flavor.
- *Oyster:* This shell-shaped mushroom has a mild, delicate flavor. Discard the knobby stem and wash the caps before using.
- *Shiitake:* This large, flat, golden-brown-capped mushroom has a woody stem. Whether you're using fresh or dried, discard the stems. Shiitakes have a pungent, woodsy flavor and are available fresh and dried. Dried shiitakes need to be soaked in warm water before use.

TOFU

Also known as bean curd, this versatile food is made from soybeans and water and either magnesium sulfate or calcium chloride as a coagulating agent.

- *Fresh tofu* is available in extra firm, firm, soft and low-fat varieties. Each one has a different texture. You can find them in the refrigerated section of most supermarkets. They are sold as 16-ounce blocks packed in water-filled plastic tubs. Both extra firm and firm tofu are ideal for grilling and stir-frying. Soft tofu is good for soup.

- *Silken tofu* comes in a foil-lined cardboard container and it has a long shelf life. You don't need to refrigerate it until it is opened. Silken tofu has a custardlike consistency. It works well for salad dressings, desserts and soups.
- *Baked seasoned tofu* is made by pressing water out of fresh tofu and baking and marinating it in seasonings or simmering it in flavored water. It has a brownish color and resilient texture. It is an ideal meat substitute in stir-fried dishes and tossed into salads. It is available in several different flavors. To make your own flavored baked tofu, see page 141.

Soymilk: The usual ingredients in soymilk are soybeans, water, sweetener and salt, and often a flavoring. This dairy-free beverage is a great alternative for those who are lactase deficient or who want to increase the amount of soy in their diet. It comes in different flavors and is easy to use in desserts and green tea beverages.

Water Chestnuts: The crunchiest of vegetables, this pale, almost translucent tuber is hard to find fresh. Canned ones are packed in water and have a mild sweet and starchy flesh. Before using, discard the water and rinse the water chestnuts in fresh water.

Wonton Wrappers: Made from wheat flour, water and sometimes eggs, these 3½-inch yellowish squares are wrapped in plastic and can be bought fresh or frozen. They can be stuffed with various fillings, then steamed or stewed in a soup. Store wrappers in the refrigerator for up to a week, or freeze for up to several months. Keep wrappers in a bag at all times to retain their moisture. When cooking with the wrappers, take out only one at a time. Leave the rest in the bag, covered with a damp cloth to prevent them from drying.

Dos for the Kitchen

+ Do wash vegetables before cutting.
+ Do wash the cutting board with soap and hot water after cutting raw meat or seafood.
+ Do dry or drain food before adding it to a heated wok or cooking pan to prevent hot oil from splattering.
+ Do apply a thin coating of oil in a wok or cooking pan to add crispness, color and flavor.
+ Do read product care instructions.
+ Do look in my cookbooks for ideas.
+ Do enjoy cooking!

Don'ts for the Kitchen

+ Don't use cooking sprays on some nonstick cookware, such as Calphalon.
+ Don't place cutting knives in the dishwasher. Wash by hand and store in a wooden block.
+ Don't leave raw foods uncovered and unrefrigerated.
+ Don't leave cooking food unattended.
+ Don't wash nonstick cookware in the dishwasher.
+ Don't use metal spatulas with nonstick cookware.
+ Don't hesitate to substitute ingredients in my recipes.
+ Don't panic when mistakes happen. See page 159, "Rescuing a Dish."

Three-Day Diet and Cleansing Program

Looking for a natural way to lose weight and cleanse your body? Try this three-day cleansing program and diet. Everything is natural, without drugs or artificial appetite suppressants. The extravaganza of soup, salad, stir-fry dishes and delicious fruit shake will taste more like gourmet meals than diet food.

Try to add soup and green tea to your daily diet. Eat them for your health, heart and well being.

Green Tea and Soup

More and more research shows that green tea and soup are secret weapons for weight loss. This three-day diet and cleansing program combines the benefits of fat-burning green tea with an increased feeling of fullness from the soup to reduce hunger and subsequent calorie intake. The large amounts of vegetables and fruit provide a rich variety of vitamins and nutrients. The vegetables and fruit cleanse your digestive system while green tea acts as a digestive aid.

Researchers recently reported in the *American Journal of Clinical Nutrition* on a six-week study conducted at the University of Geneva in Switzerland. Men taking green tea extract burned more fat calories than those taking caffeine or a placebo pill. The researchers concluded that green tea increases the rate of calorie burning beyond what can be explained by the tea's caffeine content. The researchers suggest that the caffeine combines with the natural flavonoids found in the green tea to increase basal metabolism, fat burning, or both.

Dr. Mitscher, the leading green tea researcher and author of *The Green Tea Book*, reports that

> *weight-loss experts hypothesize that green tea reduces the rate and amount of dietary carbohydrates absorbed, but without putting the body at risk of malnutrition. . . . The slow release of carbohydrates caused by green tea prevents sharp peaks of blood insulin levels, which in turn favors fat burning over fat storage.*

In recent research, the *American Society for Clinical Nutrition* reported that water incorporated into a food to make a soup, as opposed to water being served with a food, decreases calorie intake. Serving food as a soup decreases the food's caloric density while increasing the volume. This significantly increases fullness and reduces hunger and subsequent calorie intake.

Program Guidelines

It is more fun and much easier to do this program with a friend or your partner. It will positively change your attitude toward food.

Drink at least 2 quarts of purified water each day. Avoid coffee and artificial sweeteners. If you must drink coffee, drink it without cream or sweeteners.

If you are sensitive to caffeine, you can use decaffeinated green tea for drinking and cooking. Research has shown that decaffeinated green tea delivers all the health benefits of regular green tea.

If you have eaten for three days as recommended and have not cheated, you will find yourself 5 to 7 pounds lighter and more energetic than when you started. When coming off the program, eat lightly at first. Eat some light protein such as tofu, fish and chicken, then grains, before returning to a normal healthy diet.

If you want to keep the weight off and feel great forever:

+ Add tea to your daily beverage and spice rack.
+ Cut down on fat.
+ Focus on grains, fruits and vegetables.
+ Eat three regular, full meals a day.
+ Exercise, exercise, exercise.

Day 1

Drink purified water and unsweetened fruit juice. Eat as much fruit as you like, except bananas. Drink at least 2 cups of green tea on this day and eat the Green Tea–Vegetable Soup (page 37) for lunch and dinner. Enjoy the following recipes at any time: Melon Basket, without the sauce (page 171), Three-Berry Shake (page 172) and Peach Smoothie (page 173).

Day 2

Drink purified water and vegetable juice. Eat as many vegetables as you can, but no beans, peas or corn. Drink at least 2 cups of green tea on this day and eat the Green Tea–Vegetable Soup (page 37) at lunch and dinner. Enjoy the following recipes: Green Tea Sautéed Vegetables (page 127), replacing the canola oil called for in the recipes with cooking spray, Stir-Fried Bok Choy with Shiitake Mushrooms (page 129). And Spicy Green Tea Grilled Broccoli (page 131). You need to limit your oil intake for cleansing.

Day 3

Drink purified water and unsweetened fruit juice or vegetable juice. Drink at least 2 cups of green tea this day and eat the Green Tea–Vegetable Soup (page 37) with lunch and dinner. Eat dishes from Day 1 and Day 2 recipes. Reward yourself with Roasted Peppers and Potato Salad (page 125). Enjoy!

Green Tea–
Vegetable Soup

This soup is the basis of the three-day cleansing and diet program. The following portion is for one person. Eat as much soup as you can. The more you eat, the more weight you will lose. You should finish all the soup by the end of the three days. Add more water if the soup gets too dry.

6 CUPS SPRING WATER

3 GREEN TEA BAGS

5 FRESH SHIITAKE MUSHROOM CAPS, DICED

1 RED BELL PEPPER, CUT INTO 2-INCH SQUARES

½ POUND CELERY, CUT INTO 2-INCH PIECES

½ POUND CABBAGE, SHREDDED

3 TABLESPOONS MISO

¼ TEASPOON MINCED SERRANO CHILE PEPPER (OPTIONAL)

3 GREEN ONIONS (GREEN AND WHITE PARTS), MINCED

Bring the water and tea bags to a boil in a large pot.

Add the mushrooms, bell pepper, celery and cabbage and bring back to a boil. Reduce the heat to low and simmer, covered, until vegetables are tender, about 5 minutes.

Discard the tea bags. Remove ½ cup soup broth to a cup. Add the miso and stir to dissolve it in the broth.

Add the miso mixture to the remaining soup, along with the chile pepper, if using, and green onions. Simmer for 2 minutes. Serve hot. Refrigerate leftovers and reheat as needed.

Makes 7 cups

Savory Sauces and Flavorful Stocks

Sauces

A good sauce does more than add flavor to your dish. It will save you time in the kitchen. I like to make the sauces a day or two ahead, because most sauces taste much better after their flavors blend in the refrigerator overnight. Properly stored, many of the sauces will last 1 to 2 weeks. Always refrigerate them in tightly sealed containers. If using some of the sauce, use a clean dry spoon.

I have a great time making all these sauces, either alone or with friends. One weekend afternoon, I invited over two friends and had a sauce party. We doubled or tripled the recipes, and each of my friends had sauces to take home and enjoy for days or weeks. Before you begin making sauces, have plenty of small containers available. You can get them in the supermarket salad section or at cookware stores.

If a recipe calls for a sauce that you don't have on hand, don't let that stop you. Keep a supply of healthy sauces, such as those made by companies such as Eden Foods, on hand. Many of their sauces are made from organic ingredients and some are low in sodium. Don't forget to add your own personal touch when you use bottled sauces.

Stocks

Use the stocks in this chapter as the base for soups and cooking sauces.

After cooking, strain the stock and pour into a container that can be tightly sealed. The vegetables used for stock can be composted. The seafood and chicken used in making stock can be served over noodles with one of the sauces from the sauce section (pages 41–50), or as the filling for the Fresh Spring Rolls with Thai Sauce (page 80).

If you are cooking for one or two people, you can make only half of the stock recipe by simply cutting the ingredients in half.

The stock will keep refrigerated up to 5 days. Frozen, it will keep for several weeks. I like to freeze stock in ice cube trays. After the cubes are frozen, transfer them to a heavy plastic bag and seal. This makes it easy to remove only the number of cubes that you need.

Roasted Red Pepper Sauce

Use for garnishing noodle dishes or as condiment. See page 10 for ways to use the tea used for brewing the liquid.

1 CUP FRESH OR BOTTLED ROASTED RED BELL PEPPERS

½ CUP BREWED GREEN TEA (PAGE 7)

2 TABLESPOONS (ABOUT 1 OUNCE) DRY-PACKED SUN-DRIED TOMATOES, CHOPPED

2 TABLESPOONS RICE VINEGAR

2 CLOVES GARLIC, PEELED

1 TABLESPOON OLIVE OIL

½ TEASPOON WHITE PEPPER

Combine all ingredients in a blender or food processor and process until smooth. Pour into a container. Use immediately or cover and store in the refrigerator up to 1 week.

Makes 1½ cups

Spicy Sesame Sauce

This is good for dipping Fresh Spring Rolls (page 80), or as a cooking or marinade sauce. See page 10 for ways to use the liquid used for infusing the tea leaves.

1 TEASPOON WHITE SESAME SEEDS

2 CLOVES GARLIC, MINCED

1 GREEN ONION, GREEN AND WHITE PARTS,
FINELY SLICED

1 TEASPOON INFUSED GREEN TEA
LEAVES (PAGE 9), MINCED

¼ CUP TERIYAKI SAUCE

2 TABLESPOONS LEMON JUICE

1 TEASPOON SESAME OIL

1 TEASPOON THINLY SHREDDED FRESH RED CHILE PEPPER

Preheat oven to 350F (175C). Toast the sesame seeds on a baking sheet in the oven for 5 to 6 minutes, occasionally shaking the pan gently, until sesame seeds turn brown. Place in a bowl and let them cool.

Add the remaining ingredients to the sesame seeds and mix to combine. Cover and let the flavors blend in the refrigerator for about 30 minutes before using.

Makes ¾ cup

Ginger and Garlic Sauce

Use for dipping dumplings or as a marinade.

1 TEASPOON CANOLA OIL

2 TEASPOONS LOOSE GREEN TEA

¼ TABLESPOON MINCED GINGER ROOT

2 CLOVES GARLIC, MINCED

1 GREEN ONION, GREEN PART ONLY, MINCED

3 TABLESPOONS LOW-SODIUM SOY SAUCE

2 TABLESPOONS SOYMILK

2 TABLESPOONS LEMON JUICE

2 TABLESPOONS RICE VINEGAR

1 TEASPOON SESAME OIL

In a small saucepan, heat the canola oil. Add the green tea and cook, stirring, until the tea is fragrant and crispy, 10 or 20 seconds.

Combine the remaining ingredients in a small bowl. Stir in the green tea and oil. Cover and let the flavors blend in the refrigerator for 30 minutes or up to overnight.

Makes ½ cup

Spicy Cilantro Sauce

Use as a stir-fry sauce or as a marinade. See page 10 for ways to use the tea used for brewing the liquid.

4 TEASPOONS LIME JUICE

¼ CUP CHOPPED FRESH CILANTRO

4 MEDIUM CLOVES GARLIC, MINCED

2 MEDIUM GREEN ONIONS, GREEN AND
WHITE PARTS, CHOPPED

4 SMALL HOT GREEN CHILE PEPPERS,
SEEDED AND CHOPPED

2 TEASPOONS GROUND GINGER

½ TEASPOON FRESHLY GROUND WHITE PEPPER

¼ CUP BREWED GREEN TEA (PAGE 7)

2 TABLESPOONS CANOLA OIL

1 TABLESPOON FISH SAUCE

1 TEASPOON HONEY

Place all the ingredients in a blender. Process into a coarse paste. Use immediately or store in a tightly sealed container in the refrigerator for up to 1 week.

Makes ⅔ cup

Chile-Garlic Oil

This is good for stir-fry and noodle dishes, or as a garnish. Mince the chile peppers with the seeds if you want a spicier sauce. Because the oils in chile peppers are very powerful, see the tips regarding handling them.

1 TEASPOON PLUS ¼ CUP CANOLA OIL

2 TEASPOONS LOOSE GREEN TEA, PREFERABLY
GUNPOWDER OR DRAGONWELL

5 CLOVES GARLIC, MINCED

2 FRESH RED CHILE PEPPERS, MINCED

2 GREEN ONIONS, WHITE PART ONLY, MINCED

½ TEASPOON SALT

In a small saucepan, heat the 1 teaspoon oil. Add the green tea and cook, stirring, until the tea is fragrant and crispy; about 1 minute.

Place the tea, garlic, chiles, onions and salt in a short wide-mouth canning jar and mix to combine.

In the same saucepan, heat the ¼ cup oil until it is very hot. Carefully pour the hot oil over the contents of the jar. Partially cover the jar and let cool. Seal the jar tightly and store in the refrigerator for up to 2 weeks. Stir the sauce before using.

Makes ½ cup

TIPS

WEAR RUBBER GLOVES WHEN MINCING CHILE PEPPERS. TURN
THE KITCHEN FAN ON BEFORE POURING THE OIL OVER THE
CHILE MIXTURE.

Honey-Ginger Sauce

Use as a sauce or as a salad dressing. See page 10 for ways of using the tea used for brewing the liquid.

¼ CUP BREWED GREEN TEA (PAGE 7)

2 TABLESPOONS RICE VINEGAR

½ TABLESPOON HONEY

½ TABLESPOON OLIVE OIL

2 TEASPOONS FISH SAUCE

2 SMALL CLOVES GARLIC, MINCED

1 TEASPOON MINCED GINGER ROOT

1 GREEN ONION, GREEN PART ONLY, MINCED

Mix all the ingredients in a small container. Use immediately or cover and store in the refrigerator for up to 1 week.

Makes ½ cup

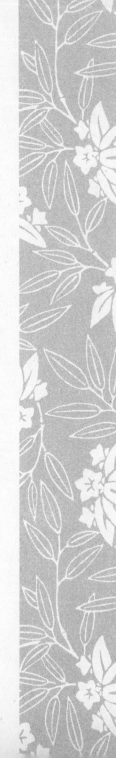

Spicy Lemon-Basil Sauce

This is good for a salad dressing, as a dipping sauce, and for cooking. Chop the chile peppers with the seeds if you want a spicier sauce. See page 10 for ways to use the tea used for brewing the liquid.

½ CUP BREWED GREEN TEA (PAGE 7)

1 TABLESPOON HONEY

2 TABLESPOONS LEMON JUICE

2 TABLESPOONS OLIVE OIL

½ CUP FRESH BASIL LEAVES, CHOPPED

2 CLOVES GARLIC, CHOPPED

1 SMALL JALAPEÑO CHILE PEPPER, CHOPPED

¼ TEASPOON SALT

¼ TEASPOON WHITE PEPPER

Combine all the ingredients in a blender and process until pureed. Pour into a container and use immediately or cover and store in the refrigerator for up to 2 weeks.

Makes 1 cup

Curry Peanut Sauce

Use for dipping spring rolls or as a sauce for noodles.

1 TABLESPOON CANOLA OIL

CONTENTS OF 1 BAG GREEN TEA

2 CLOVES GARLIC, MINCED

1 TEASPOON GRATED GINGER ROOT

¼ CUP MINCED ONION

½ CUP REDUCED-FAT PEANUT BUTTER

½ CUP SOYMILK

½ TABLESPOON LEMON JUICE

1 TEASPOON CURRY POWDER

In a small saucepan, heat the oil over medium heat. Add the green tea, garlic, ginger and onion and sauté until the onion softens, 4 to 5 minutes.

Add the peanut butter, soymilk, lemon juice and curry powder. Cook, stirring, until the sauce is hot and the peanut butter melts, 1 to 2 minutes.

Let the sauce cool. Use immediately or store in the refrigerator in a tightly sealed container for up to 1 week.

Makes about 1½ cups

TIP

FOR A SMOOTHER SAUCE, PROCESS IN A BLENDER FOR 20 SECONDS.

Green Tea–Ginger Sauce

This is good with seafood. See page 10 for ways to use the tea used for brewing the liquid.

½ CUP BREWED GREEN TEA (PAGE 7)

¼ CUP FINELY SHREDDED GINGER ROOT

¼ CUP RICE WINE OR DRY SHERRY

¼ CUP RICE VINEGAR

1 TABLESPOON FISH SAUCE

1 TEASPOON SESAME OIL

1 SMALL GREEN ONION, GREEN AND
WHITE PARTS, MINCED

4 CLOVES GARLIC, MINCED

½ TEASPOON MINCED RED CHILE PEPPER (OPTIONAL)

Mix all the ingredients in a small container. Use immediately, or cover and store in the refrigerator for up to 2 weeks.

Makes 1 cup

Thai Sauce

Use for dipping, as a salad or as a cooking sauce. Page 10 gives
ways to use the tea used for brewing the liquid.

1 TEASPOON CANOLA OIL

1 SMALL FRESH RED CHILE PEPPER, MINCED

2 CLOVES GARLIC, MINCED

½ CUP BREWED GREEN TEA (PAGE 7)

1 TABLESPOON HONEY

¼ CUP RICE VINEGAR

1 TABLESPOON FISH SAUCE

Heat the oil in a small saucepan over medium-high
heat. Add the chile and garlic and sauté till fragrant,
about 30 seconds. Add the green tea, honey, vinegar,
and fish sauce. Bring to a boil, and remove from heat.

Let the sauce cool. Use immediately or store in a
tightly sealed container in the refrigerator for up to
1 week.

Makes 1 cup

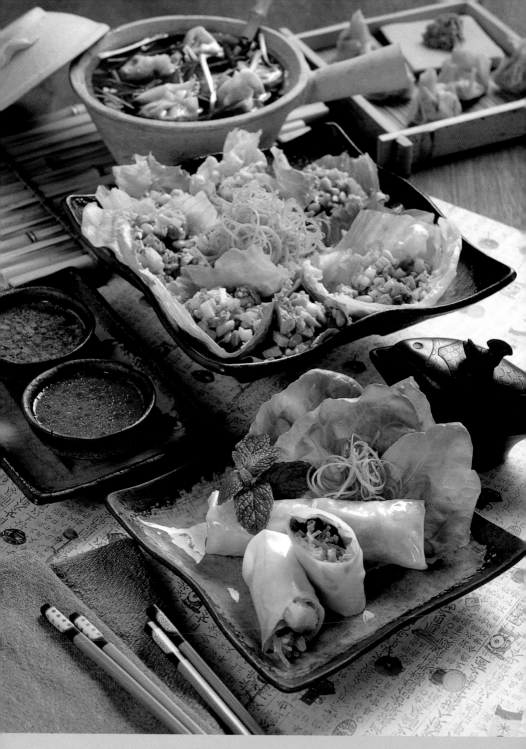

Wontons (top right); Shiitake Mushroom–Wonton Soup (top left);
Flavored Tofu in Lettuce Cups (center); Thai Sauce, Honey-Ginger
Sauce (center left, front and back); Fresh Spring Rolls (bottom).

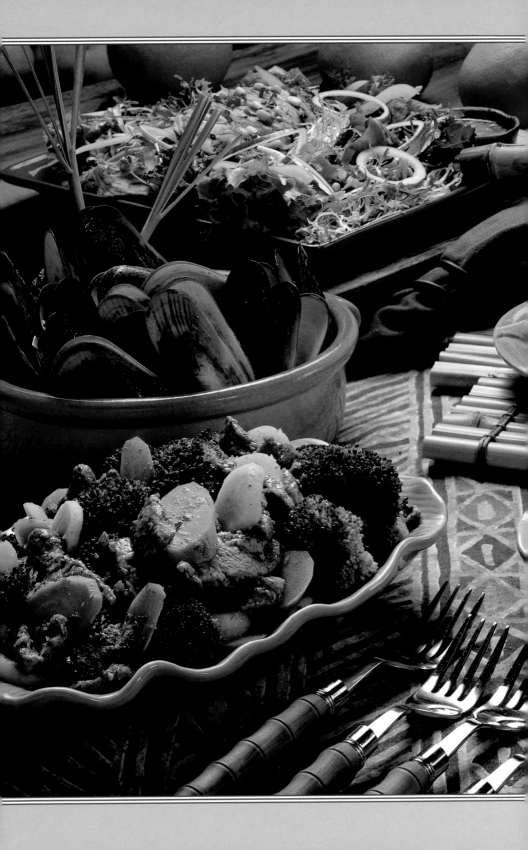

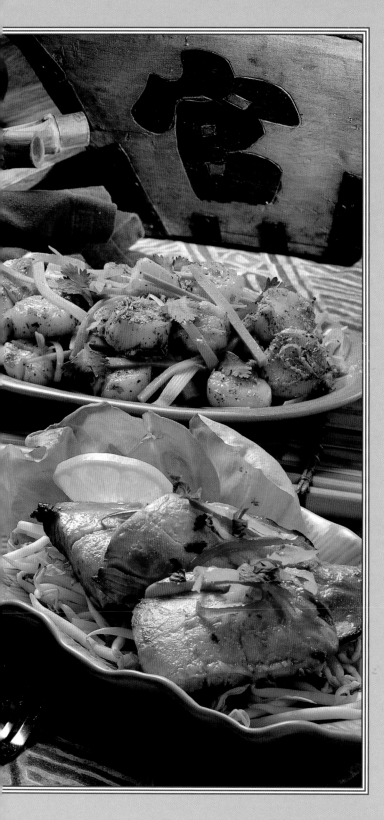

CLOCKWISE FROM TOP LEFT: Spicy and Colorful Chicken Salad; Orange-Flavored Scallops; Green-Tea-and-Orange-Smoked Salmon; Lemon and Ginger Pork with Vegetables; Mussels in Lemon Grass–Green Tea Wine Sauce.

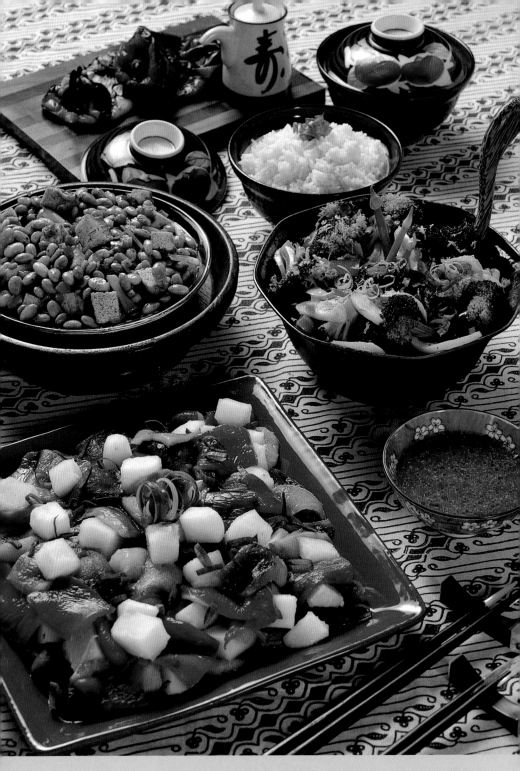

CLOCKWISE FROM TOP LEFT: Shelled Green Soybeans with Baked Tofu;
Green Tea–Sautéed Vegetables; Thai Sauce; Roasted Peppers and Potato Salad.

Green Tea–Vegetable Stock

With a delicious stock on hand, dishes such as soups can be made quickly. Use this not only for soups but also for stir-frying, or even substitute it for the water when cooking rice for flavored steamed rice.

6 BAGS GREEN TEA

8 CUPS BOILING WATER

2 TABLESPOONS CANOLA OIL

2 TABLESPOONS (½-INCH) GINGER ROOT CHUNKS

1 CUP FRESH OYSTER OR SHIITAKE MUSHROOMS, MINCED

1 FRESH RED CHILE PEPPER, MINCED

5 GREEN ONIONS, TRIMMED AND CUT DIAGONALLY INTO 1-INCH-LONG SHREDS

20 BABY CARROTS, CUT DIAGONALLY INTO ¼-INCH CHUNKS

2 CUPS (¼-INCH) TOMATO CUBES

1 CUP FRESH OR FROZEN WHOLE-KERNEL CORN

SALT AND WHITE PEPPER, TO TASTE

2 TEASPOONS SESAME OIL

Place the green tea bags in a large pot. Add the boiling water and simmer over low heat for 3 minutes. Use a spoon to press the tea out of the tea bags. Discard the tea bags.

Heat the oil in a nonstick wok or chef's pan over medium-high heat and swirl to coat pan. Add the ginger, mushrooms, chile and green onions and stir-fry for 1 minute. Add the carrots, tomatoes and corn. Cover and cook, stirring occasionally, until the carrots soften, about 2 minutes.

Add the vegetable mixture to the tea and bring the mixture to a boil. Reduce the heat and simmer, covered, for 40 minutes. Season with salt and white pepper. Stir in the sesame oil.

Strain the liquid through a colander, pressing out as much liquid as possible. Let cool. Pour stock into a container and refrigerate or freeze (page 40).

Makes about 5 to 6 cups

Green Tea–Seafood Stock

Traditionally, seafood stock called for fish heads and bones, which require hours of cooking. I have developed this simple and healthy seafood stock which I cook with many of my favorite dishes.

6 GREEN TEA BAGS

8 CUPS BOILING WATER

2 TABLESPOONS CANOLA OIL

2 TABLESPOONS (¼-INCH) GINGER ROOT CHUNKS

4 CLOVES GARLIC, QUARTERED

1 CUP FRESH OYSTER OR SHIITAKE MUSHROOMS, MINCED

1 FRESH RED CHILE PEPPER, MINCED

2 MEDIUM LEEKS, WHITE PART ONLY, CUT DIAGONALLY INTO ½-INCH CHUNKS

½ POUND SCALLOPS

½ POUND FRESH OR FROZEN WHITE FISH FILLET, CUT INTO 2-INCH PIECES

12 SPRIGS FRESH CILANTRO

1 TEASPOON WHITE PEPPER

Place the green tea bags in a large pot. Add the boiling water and simmer over low heat for 3 minutes. Use a spoon to press the tea out of the tea bags. Discard the tea bags.

Heat a wok or chef's pan over medium heat and coat it with the oil. Add the ginger, garlic, mush-

rooms, chile and leeks, and sauté until the leeks
soften and become fragrant, about 2 minutes.

Add the vegetable mixture to the tea and bring
the mixture to a boil. Add the scallops, fish and
cilantro. Return to a boil. Reduce the heat and simmer, covered, for 40 minutes. Season with white pepper.

Strain the liquid through a colander, pressing out
as much liquid as possible. Let cool. Pour stock into a
container and refrigerate or freeze (page 40).

Makes 5 to 6 cups

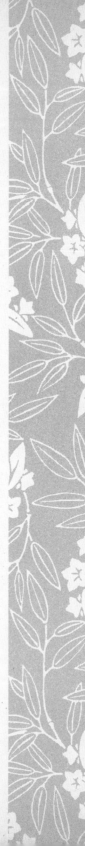

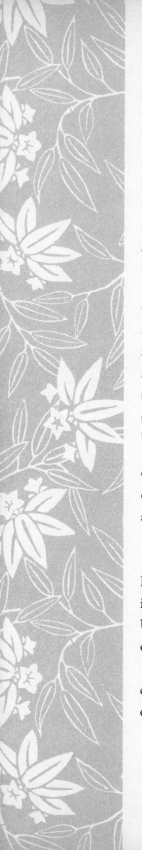

Green Tea–
Chicken Stock

Many chicken stock recipes call for chicken bones or the whole chicken, which require 4 or 5 hours to cook. I have come up this healthy and simple way to make the chicken stock. This stock not only has less fat and takes less time than traditional recipes but is more flavorful than the commercial brands.

6 BAGS GREEN TEA

2 CUPS BOILING WATER

2 TABLESPOONS CANOLA OIL

2 TABLESPOONS (½-INCH) GINGER ROOT CHUNKS

5 CLOVES GARLIC, MINCED

5 GREEN ONIONS, TRIMMED AND CUT INTO 1-INCH-LONG
PIECES

1 POUND SKINLESS CHICKEN BREAST, CUT INTO 1-INCH
CHUNKS

6 CUPS CANNED CHICKEN BROTH

3 CUPS FRESH OR FROZEN WHOLE-KERNEL CORN

1 TEASPOON WHITE PEPPER

Place the green tea bags in a large pot. Add the boiling water and simmer over low heat for 3 minutes. Use a spoon to press the tea out of the tea bags. Discard the tea leaves.

Heat a wok or chef's pan over medium heat and coat it with the oil. Add the ginger, garlic and green onions and sauté until fragrant, about 1 minute. Add the chicken. Sauté till the chicken browns, 2 to 3 minutes.

Add the chicken mixture, chicken broth and corn to the tea. Bring to a boil. Reduce the heat and simmer, covered, for 40 minutes. Season with white pepper.

Strain the liquid through a colander, pressing out as much liquid as possible. Let cool. Pour stock into a container and refrigerate or freeze (page 40).

Makes 5 to 6 cups

Warming Soups and Appealing Appetizers

Soups

Are you amazed over the number of canned soups on the market? Many of them are high in fat and sodium and have been sitting on the shelves for weeks.

What about freshly homemade, nurturing soups? They don't have to be a rare offering. With a good pot and a few fresh ingredients you can make soup that warms your heart and kitchen. Homemade soups will calm your mind and soothe your spirit.

The keys to tasty homemade soup are the stock and the combination of ingredients. Use one of the homemade stocks with green tea (pages 51–56) or a good commercial stock as a base for your soup. Different stocks and ingredients give each soup its own personality, making the variety of soups limitless.

With a good stock, you no longer have to spend hours in your kitchen watching the soup simmer to develop a rich flavor. With fresh, fast-cooking ingredients and a good stock, most of the soups, such as Tofu and Spinach Miso Soup and Soup from the Sea, require only a few minutes to make. Many of them make a light meal on their own, such as Shiitake Mushroom–Wonton Soup and Chicken Noodle Soup.

To round out a bowl of soup, serve it with bread, salad or appetizers.

Appetizers

Many popular appetizers are deep-fried and are high in fat. If you overindulge on them, you are too full for your main course. I have tried to develop luscious, healthy appetizers that don't use up your daily fat allowance and cause you to lose enthusiasm for your next course. You will find unusual dishes such as Braised Stuffed Shiitake Mushrooms, Pearl Rice Balls, Stuffed Cucumbers with Thai Sauce and Marble Eggs.

Be creative with appetizers and combine and match them with other dishes. Don't limit appetizers to just a starter or finger food at a party. Almond Butter Rolls, Fresh Spring Rolls with Thai Sauce, and Creative Dumpling Delight can be served as a meal in themselves.

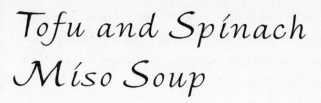

Tofu and Spinach Miso Soup

Many Asians start the day with miso soup. To maximize the benefits of the soy protein from the miso, blend the miso paste and broth well. Don't overcook the soup once the miso is added. This will destroy some of the nutritional value. See page 10 for ways to use the tea used to brew the liquid.

2 CUPS BREWED GREEN TEA (PAGE 7)

2 CUPS VEGETABLE STOCK (PAGE 51 OR PURCHASED)

4 SLICES GINGER ROOT, EACH THE SIZE OF A QUARTER

1 (12-OZ.) PACKAGE FIRM SILKEN TOFU, CUT INTO ½-INCH CUBES

2 TABLESPOONS MISO

2 CUPS PACKED SPINACH LEAVES, LARGE STEMS REMOVED

2 TEASPOONS SESAME OIL

½ CUP CHOPPED GREEN ONIONS

LOW-SODIUM SOY SAUCE, TO TASTE

In a large saucepan, bring the green tea, stock and ginger to a boil.

Add the tofu. Bring back to a boil. Reduce heat, cover, and simmer until tofu is heated through, 2 or 3 minutes.

Remove about ½ cup of the broth to a bowl. Add the miso, and stir into a smooth, thin paste. Pour the paste back into the soup and add the spinach. Bring

back to a boil. Stir in sesame oil. Remove from heat and ladle into bowls. Sprinkle with sesame oil and green onions. Soy sauce may be passed at the table if desired. Serve hot.

Makes 4 servings

Soup from the Sea

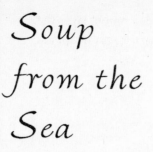

I served this dish to friends who claimed that they didn't like seafood or soup. They not only ate all the soup, but left with the recipe. Sometimes the sunflower sprouts are hard to find, but they are definitely worth the search. I can always find them at the health food store. See page 10 for ways to use the tea used to brew the liquid.

2 CUPS BREWED GREEN TEA (PAGE 7)

2 CUPS GREEN TEA–SEAFOOD STOCK (PAGE 53)

4 SLICES GINGER, EACH THE SIZE OF A QUARTER

4 (ABOUT 4-INCH-SQUARE) PIECES TOASTED NORI

½ POUND MEDIUM SHRIMP, SHELLED AND DEVEINED

½ POUND MEDIUM SCALLOPS

2 CUPS SUNFLOWER SPROUTS OR BEAN SPROUTS

SALT AND WHITE PEPPER, TO TASTE

1 TEASPOON SESAME OIL

2 GREEN ONIONS, GREEN AND WHITE PARTS, MINCED

In a large saucepan, bring the green tea, stock, ginger and nori to a boil.

Add shrimp and scallops and bring back to a boil. Reduce heat, cover, and simmer for 3 minutes.

Add the sprouts and bring back to a boil; don't overcook the sprouts. Season with salt and pepper.

Sprinkle the sesame oil and green onions over the soup and serve hot.

Makes 4 servings

VARIATION

FOR A SPICY SOUP, ADD 1 TEASPOON CHILE-GARLIC OIL (PAGE 45) WITH THE SALT AND PEPPER.

Broccoli Soup with Yogurt

Did you know that broccoli is rich in calcium? This is a vital mineral for women, who need it to keep their bones strong. Researchers also believe that broccoli may help prevent cancer, protect against heart disease and boost the immune system. See page 10 for ways to use the tea used to brew the liquid.

2 TEASPOONS CANOLA OIL

4 CLOVES GARLIC, MINCED

½ JALAPEÑO CHILE PEPPER, SEEDED AND MINCED
(OPTIONAL)

1 LEEK, WHITE PART ONLY, FINELY CHOPPED

2 CUPS BREWED GREEN TEA (PAGE 7)

2 CUPS VEGETABLE STOCK (PAGE 51
OR PURCHASED)

3 CUPS BROCCOLI FLORETS

¼ CUP RICE MILK OR SOYMILK

2 TABLESPOONS FRESH MINT LEAVES, MINCED

SALT AND WHITE PEPPER, TO TASTE

½ CUP PLAIN YOGURT

Heat the oil in a large nonstick pot over medium-high heat. Add the garlic and jalapeño. Stir-fry until brown, about 1 minute. Add the leek and stir-fry over medium heat until leek softens, 2 to 3 minutes. Stir in the green tea and stock and simmer for 10 minutes.

While the soup simmers, cook the broccoli in

rapidly boiling water until bright green, about 1 minute. Drain the broccoli in a colander and rinse under water to set the color. Drain.

In a blender, puree the soup, in batches, with the broccoli, rice milk and mint. Return the soup to the pot and heat thoroughly. Season with salt and pepper. Serve lukewarm or chilled. Garnish each serving with a dollop of yogurt.

Makes 5 or 6 servings

Shiitake Mushroom– Wonton Soup

I like to make my wontons nice and plump, twice as big as the restaurant ones. Wontons freeze very well. To freeze: First, place them on a lightly floured plate with enough space between them so they don't touch. Put the plate in your freezer until the wontons are frozen solid. Then remove them from the plate and seal them in a plastic bag. To cook the frozen wontons, drop them into boiling soup and cook them a little longer than fresh ones. See page 10 for ways to use the tea used to brew the liquid.

6 DRIED SHIITAKE MUSHROOMS

24 WONTON WRAPPERS

4 CUPS CHICKEN STOCK (PAGE 55
OR PURCHASED, FAT-FREE)

2 CUPS BREWED GREEN TEA (PAGE 7)

1 TEASPOON SESAME OIL

⅛ TEASPOON WHITE PEPPER

2 GREEN ONIONS, GREEN PART ONLY, SHREDDED

SHREDDED RED BELL PEPPER, FOR GARNISH

WONTON FILLING

4 TEASPOONS LOOSE GREEN TEA

¼ POUND LARGE RAW SHRIMP, FINELY CHOPPED

¼ POUND EXTRA LEAN GROUND PORK OR CHICKEN BREAST

1 TEASPOON SESAME OIL

1 TABLESPOON LOW-SODIUM SOY SAUCE

1 TEASPOON CANOLA OIL

2 TEASPOONS MINCED FRESH GINGER ROOT

2 CLOVES GARLIC, MINCED

¼ CUP CANNED WATER CHESTNUTS, FINELY CHOPPED

2 TEASPOONS RICE VINEGAR

Soak the mushrooms in warm water until softened, about 15 minutes. Rinse the undersides of the soaked mushrooms under cold running water to clean them of any dirt or sand. Squeeze the mushrooms in your hand to thoroughly wring out the water. Discard the stems and thinly shred the caps.

Make the filling: Steep the tea in ½ cup boiling water for 5 minutes and drain. Mince the tea leaves. (See page 10 for ways to use the liquid.) In a large bowl, combine the shrimp, pork, tea leaves, sesame oil and soy sauce. Mix well; set aside. Heat the canola oil in a nonstick saucepan over medium-high heat. Add the ginger, garlic and water chestnuts and stir-fry until fragrant, about 1 minute. Add the rice vinegar. Add to the shrimp and pork mixture and stir to combine.

Dip all edges of a wonton wrapper in a bowl of cold water. Place 1 tablespoon filling in the center of the wrapper. Pinch edges to seal. Repeat with remaining wrappers and filling. Cover the filled wontons and remaining wrappers with moistened towels to prevent drying.

Place the stock, green tea and mushrooms in a large pot. Bring to a boil. Add the wontons, stirring gently to prevent wontons from sticking to the bottom of the pot. Wontons will float to the top when

done, 3 to 5 minutes. Stir in the sesame oil and white pepper.

Ladle the wontons and broth into 6 deep soup bowls. Garnish each with the green onions and bell pepper. Serve hot.

Makes 6 servings

Chicken Noodle Soup

In this soup, the green tea–marinated chicken is paired with rice noodles. The soup is fresh and cooling. This nurturing dish is ideal for a cold winter day, a new mother or a sick friend. Bean thread noodles can be quite slippery, challenging your skill with chopsticks, so keep a fork handy. See page 10 for ways to use the tea used to brew the liquid.

8 OUNCES BONELESS, SKINLESS CHICKEN BREAST, CUT INTO ½-INCH CHUNKS

½ CUP BREWED GREEN TEA (PAGE 7)

5 OUNCES DRY BEAN THREAD NOODLES

4 CUPS CHICKEN STOCK (PAGE 55 OR PURCHASED, FAT-FREE)

2 (½-INCH-THICK) SLICES GINGER ROOT, LIGHTLY MASHED

½ CUP OYSTER MUSHROOMS, CUBED

3 CUPS PACKED SPINACH LEAVES, LARGE STEMS REMOVED

SALT AND WHITE PEPPER, TO TASTE

1 TABLESPOON FRESH MINT LEAVES OR CILANTRO LEAVES

Place the chicken in a large bowl and add the green tea. Cover and refrigerate 1 hour to marinate.

Cover the bean thread noodles with warm water. Soak until softened, about 10 minutes. Drain.

In a big pot, bring the stock, ginger, and mushrooms to a boil over high heat. Reduce heat and sim-

mer for 2 minutes. Add the chicken, including the tea marinade, and noodles. Return to a boil. Reduce heat and simmer for 3 minutes. Add the spinach and boil for 2 minutes. Season with salt and pepper. Ladle into bowl and garnish with mint leaves.

Makes 4 to 6 servings

VARIATION

FOR A SPICY VERSION, SERVE WITH THAI SAUCE (PAGE 50).

Flavored Tofu in Lettuce Cups

Because you can almost see through lettuce leaves, the Chinese call lettuce the glass vegetable. It is considered a delicate vegetable and often served on festive occasions. A dish that I ate at a banquet in Beijing was my inspiration for this one.

¼ CUP CANOLA OIL

2 TEASPOONS MINCED GINGER ROOT

1 TABLESPOON LOOSE GREEN TEA, PREFERABLY
GUNPOWDER

1 CUP OYSTER MUSHROOMS, FINELY CHOPPED

8 OUNCES FLAVORED BAKED TOFU (PAGE 141
OR PURCHASED), FINELY CHOPPED INTO CUBES

½ CUP FINELY CUBED CARROT

½ CUP FINELY CUBED GREEN APPLE

½ CUP WATER CHESTNUTS, FINELY CHOPPED INTO
CUBES

¼ CUP GINGER AND GARLIC SAUCE (PAGE 43)

SALT AND BLACK PEPPER, TO TASTE

½ CUP PINE NUTS, TOASTED (PAGE 124)

1 TEASPOON SESAME OIL

2 GREEN ONIONS, GREEN PART ONLY, MINCED

24 SMALL ICEBERG LETTUCE CUPS

HONEY-GINGER SAUCE (PAGE 46), TO SERVE

Heat the oil in a nonstick wok or cooking pan over medium-high heat and swirl to coat. Add the ginger and tea and stir-fry until fragrant, about 30 seconds.

Add the mushrooms and tofu and stir-fry for 2 minutes. Add the carrot, apple and water chestnuts and stir-fry for 30 seconds.

Add the Ginger and Garlic Sauce. Cook, stirring occasionally, until vegetables and apple are heated through, about 2 minutes. Season with salt and pepper. Add the pine nuts, sesame oil and green onions and toss to combine.

To serve, spoon 2 tablespoons of the mixture into a lettuce cup, wrap and eat out of your hand. Serve with the Honey-Ginger Sauce.

Makes 24 appetizers

Braised Stuffed Shiitake Mushrooms

Shiitake mushrooms are very popular in Asia. Vendors sell them fresh or dried on the street the way ice cream or hot dogs are sold in the United States, except that they are much healthier. Not only are they an important source of nutrients, but also research suggests that they may fight cancer, lower cholesterol and stimulate the immune system.

20 MEDIUM FRESH OR DRIED SHIITAKE MUSHROOMS

WONTON FILLING (PAGE 45)

SPICY LEMON-BASIL SAUCE (PAGE 47) OR ROASTED RED PEPPER SAUCE (PAGE 41), TO SERVE

For fresh mushrooms, wash and discard the stems. For dried mushrooms, soak the mushrooms in warm tea until softened, about 15 minutes. Rinse the undersides of the soaked mushrooms under cold running water to clean them of any dirt or sand. Squeeze the mushrooms in your hand to thoroughly wring out the water. Discard the stems.

Make the filling. Preheat the broiler.

Place mushroom caps, stem sides up, in a greased baking pan. Spoon 1 tablespoon of the

filling mixture into each cap. Spray lightly with cooking spray.

Broil with the tops 4 inches from heat 5 to 7 minutes, until shrimp mixture is light brown. Serve hot with sauce.

Makes 20 appetizers

Pearl Rice Balls

Glutinous rice gets its sticky character from its high starch content. It gives the appearance of translucent pearls on the outside of these meatballs. The green tea gives these "pearl" balls a distinctive flavor. They can be prepared ahead of time, then covered and refrigerated for up to 2 days. Heat in a steamer or microwave before serving. When I serve this dish at parties, they disappear so fast!

If using the shiitake mushrooms, discard the stems, but use the stems of oyster mushrooms.

1½ CUPS UNCOOKED GLUTINOUS RICE

4 BAGS GREEN TEA

1 POUND FRESH SPINACH, LARGE STEMS REMOVED

ROASTED RED PEPPER SAUCE (PAGE 41), TO SERVE

FILLING

1 POUND EXTRA LEAN GROUND PORK

2 FRESH SHIITAKE OR OYSTER MUSHROOMS, MINCED

CONTENTS OF 2 BAGS GREEN TEA

4 GREEN ONIONS, CHOPPED

1 TABLESPOON MINCED GINGER ROOT

2 TEASPOONS CHOPPED FRESH CILANTRO

1 TABLESPOON SESAME OIL

1 TEASPOON WHITE PEPPER

3 TABLESPOONS LOW-SODIUM SOY SAUCE

Cover the rice with cold water in a large bowl. Let stand 2 hours.

Make the filling: Place all the filling ingredients in a large bowl and mix well. Drain rice and place it in a bowl.

With wet hands, roll filling mixture into balls, using about 1 tablespoon for each. Roll each meatball in rice until coated.

Line a steamer rack or a heatproof plate with wet cheesecloth. Arrange meatballs, without crowding, on cheesecloth.

In a large pot, bring 5 to 6 cups water to a boil. Add the tea bags. Place the meatballs over the boiling tea. Cover and steam over high heat until pork is no longer pink and rice is tender, 15 to 20 minutes. Set steamer rack with meatballs aside.

Add the spinach to the tea and boil until bright green, about 20 seconds. Drain well.

Line the serving plate with the spinach. Arrange the meatballs on top. Serve hot with the sauce.

Makes 35 appetizers

Almond Butter Rolls

The rolls can be made up to 2 hours ahead of time but will taste best if you serve them when they are still warm. See page 10 for ways to use the tea used to brew the liquid.

1 CARROT, SHREDDED

1 CUCUMBER, SHREDDED

½ RED BELL PEPPER, SHREDDED

4 (10-INCH) FLOUR TORTILLAS

4 TABLESPOONS CREAMY ALMOND BUTTER OR
PEANUT BUTTER

ROASTED RED PEPPER SAUCE (PAGE 41)

MARINADE

2 CUPS COLD BREWED GREEN TEA (PAGE 7)

2 TABLESPOONS RICE VINEGAR

1 TABLESPOON WHITE PEPPER

Make the marinade: Combine all the ingredients in a medium bowl. Add the carrot, cucumber, and bell pepper and marinate for 30 minutes. Drain well.

Warm the tortillas in a microwave on high for 30 seconds, or warm on a baking sheet in a 350F (175C) oven about 2 minutes, or until soft, or steam them briefly in a steamer. Store the warm tortillas between wet paper towels in a covered dish.

Lay 1 tortilla flat on a work surface. Spread with 1 tablespoon of the almond butter. Top with one-

fourth of the vegetables. Tightly roll the tortillas up to make thick tubes. Cut each roll into four equal pieces. Serve warm with sauce.

Makes 16 appetizers

TIP

TO STORE THE ROLLS, COVER WITH WET PAPER TOWELS AND
PLACE IN A PLASTIC BAG. WARM THE ROLLS BEFORE SERVING.

Stuffed Cucumbers with Spicy Lemon-Basil Sauce

If you like a vegetarian version, substitute firm tofu for the chicken. You can always double or triple the filling and freeze the extra portion for the next occasion.

6 ENGLISH CUCUMBERS, EACH AT LEAST 8 INCHES
LONG AND 2 INCHES IN DIAMETER

4 BAGS GREEN TEA

SPICY LEMON-BASIL SAUCE (PAGE 47) OR GINGER
AND GARLIC SAUCE (PAGE 43)

FILLING

¼ POUND EXTRA LEAN GROUND CHICKEN OR PORK

½ CUP CHOPPED CANNED WATER CHESTNUTS

3 MEDIUM FRESH OR DRIED SHIITAKE MUSHROOMS, MINCED

3 MEDIUM GREEN ONIONS, GREEN AND WHITE PARTS,
CHOPPED

1 TABLESPOON MINCED GINGER ROOT

2 CLOVES GARLIC, MINCED

2 TABLESPOONS GINGER AND GARLIC SAUCE (PAGE 43)

Make the filling: Combine all ingredients in a medium bowl. Set the filling aside while preparing the cucumbers.

Peel the cucumbers and trim off both ends. Cut each cucumber crosswise into 5 sections. Remove the seeds and pith with an apple corer or a small knife.

Stuff the cucumber pieces with 1 tablespoon of the filling mixture. Arrange the rounds in 2 shallow 8-inch dishes or whatever dishes will fit in your steamer.

In a large pot, bring 4 cups water to a boil. Add the tea bags. Place one of the dishes over the boiling tea. Cover and steam over medium-high heat until the filling is no longer pink, 12 to 15 minutes. Repeat with remaining dish. Serve warm with sauce.

Makes 30 appetizers

Fresh Spring Rolls with Thai Sauce

I never had a birthday cake while growing up in China. Since I loved these rolls and my birthday is near the beginning of spring, my mother would make them for my birthday parties.

Page 10 gives uses for the tea used to brew the liquid.

12 (8-INCH) ROUND DRIED RICE PAPER WRAPPERS

24 COOKED MEDIUM SHRIMP, SHELLED AND DEVEINED

24 FRESH BASIL LEAVES OR MINT LEAVES

FILLING

2 OUNCES DRIED THIN BEAN THREAD NOODLES

2 CUPS HOT BREWED GREEN TEA (PAGE 7)

4 GREEN ONIONS, GREEN PART ONLY, CUT INTO SHORT THIN SLIVERS

1 MEDIUM RED BELL PEPPER, CUT INTO SHORT THIN STRIPS

2 CUPS COLD BREWED GREEN TEA (PAGE 7)

½ TABLESPOON SESAME OIL

1 TABLESPOON THAI SAUCE (PAGE 50)

SALT AND WHITE PEPPER, TO TASTE

DIPPING SAUCE

½ CUP THAI SAUCE (PAGE 50)

Make the filling: Cover the bean thread noodles with the hot green tea and soak until softened, about 15 minutes; drain. Cut into 3-inch lengths. In a bowl, soak the green onions and bell pepper in the cold tea for 20 minutes. Drain.

Place all the filling ingredients in a bowl. Stir lightly to mix.

Soak a sheet of rice paper in warm water until soft, about 1 minute. Carefully transfer the rice paper to a dry cutting board.

Arrange 2 shrimp, side by side, in a row along the bottom third of the rice paper. Place one basil leaf on top of each shrimp and top with 2 to 3 tablespoons of the filling. Roll up the rice paper to form a tight cylinder, folding in the side about halfway, as you would to form an egg roll or a blintz. Assemble the remaining spring rolls the same way. Cut each spring roll in half on the diagonal. Serve with dipping sauce.

Makes 12 rolls

Creative Dumpling Delight

When people find out I'm from China, they often ask, "Is green tea really that good for you?" When they find out I write cookbooks, they're likely to ask, "So you know how to make dumplings?" Even better, I know how to make dumplings with green tea.

40 SQUARE WONTON WRAPPERS

40 LARGE THIN CARROT ROUNDS (ABOUT 2 THICK CARROTS)

6 BAGS GREEN TEA

GINGER AND GARLIC SAUCE (PAGE 43)

FILLING

2 TEASPOONS CANOLA OIL

1 TABLESPOON MINCED GINGER ROOT

1 CUP MINCED LEEKS

¾ POUND EXTRA-LEAN GROUND PORK

1 TABLESPOON RICE WINE

¼ TEASPOON PEPPER

DASH OF SALT

Make the filling: Heat the oil in a small nonstick skillet over medium-high heat. Add the ginger and sauté until lightly browned, about 1 minute. Add the leeks and sauté until softened, about 2 minutes.

Combine the leeks with the remaining filling ingredients in a large bowl. Mix well.

Set up a space for folding the dumplings. Place a bowl of cold water, the wonton wrappers, the filling and a steamer basket around your work area. Cover the wrappers with a damp paper towel to prevent drying. Arrange the carrot rounds in the steamer.

With each wrapper, dip all four edges into the cold water. Holding the wrapper flat on your palm, place about 1 heaping teaspoon of the filling in the center. Bring the four corners of the wrapper up over the filling. Pinch the edges together tightly. Set each dumpling on a carrot round. Leave a little space between the dumplings.

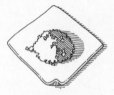

1. Dip the edges of the wrapper in water. Place a heaping teaspoon of filling in the center.
2. Bring up the four corners over the filling.
3. Pinch the edges together to seal.

In a large pot, bring 4 to 5 cups of water to a boil. Add the tea bags. Place the dumplings over the boiling tea. Make sure the water doesn't reach the dumplings. Cover and steam over high heat until dumpling skins are translucent, 10 to 12 minutes. Serve warm with sauce.

Makes 40 dumplings

TIPS

THERE SHOULD BE ADEQUATE WATER IN THE POT FOR SEV-
ERAL MINUTES OF BOILING, BUT IT SHOULD NOT TOUCH THE
DUMPLINGS IN THE STEAMER. IF YOU DON'T HAVE A STEAMER
BASKET, YOU CAN USE A HEATPROOF PLATE. PUT A HEAT-
PROOF BOWL ON THE BOTTOM OF THE POT. ADD WATER AND
TEA TO THE POT. FILL THE BOWL WITH WATER AND PLACE THE
PLATE ON TOP. COVER AND STEAM.

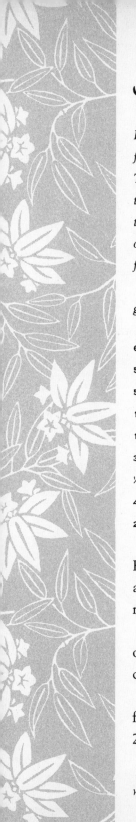

Marble Eggs

In China, this is the best-known dish cooked with tea. The tea flavor and color seeps through the cracked shells into the eggs. The result is stunning. After you taste this, you may never want to eat plain hard-cooked eggs again. The longer the eggs soak in the sauce the more flavorful they become. Marble eggs are not only good as a garnish but are ideal as a snack or lunch box filler.

As a child I loved to gather eggs from the nests of my grandmother's chickens so that she could make this dish for me.

6 EGGS

5 CUPS WATER

5 BAGS GREEN TEA

1 TEASPOON BLACK PEPPER

1 (1-INCH) CINNAMON STICK

3 TABLESPOONS LOW-SODIUM SOY SAUCE

½ TEASPOON FIVE-SPICE POWDER

4 THIN SLICES GINGER ROOT

2 DRIED RED CHILE PEPPERS (OPTIONAL)

Place eggs in a large saucepan. Cover with cold water and bring to a boil over high heat. Reduce heat to medium and cook 7 minutes.

With the back of a large spoon, lightly tap eggs over the entire shell to produce a spider web of cracks. Do not peel. Return eggs to water.

Add tea bags, pepper, cinnamon stick, soy sauce, five-spice powder, ginger and chiles, if using. Boil for 2 minutes. Reduce heat to low. Cover and simmer 40 to 50 minutes. Let eggs stay in the sauce until serving time. Peel the eggs and remove any membrane before serving. Serve sliced, quartered, or whole at room temperature or chilled.

Makes 6 eggs

Pan-Fried Garlic Scallop Dumplings

These dumplings serve well as a starter or can stand on their own as a snack. Traditionally, the dumplings are pan-fried with large amounts of oil. Using less oil and water to pan-fry the dumplings makes them crisp on the bottom and tender on top, but without the extra fat.

If you would like to impress your guests and save time, you can use the gyoza pack (a handy gadget to fold and seal dumplings, which creates pretty ruffled edges) to make the dumpling. Remember that the most important thing is not the look of the dumpling but having your wrappers and filling stay together until you eat them. Serve hot with Ginger and Garlic Sauce (page 43).

40 ROUND (GYOZA) DUMPLING WRAPPERS

2 TABLESPOONS CANOLA OIL

½ CUP WATER

SLICED GREEN ONIONS (OPTIONAL)

EDIBLE FLOWERS (OPTIONAL)

½ TEASPOON CHILE-GARLIC OIL (PAGE 45) OR SPICY SESAME SAUCE (PAGE 42)

FILLING

4 TEASPOONS LOOSE GREEN TEA

½ POUND FRESH SEA SCALLOPS, MINCED

¼ CUP ONION, MINCED

4 CLOVES GARLIC, MINCED

1 TABLESPOON MINCED GINGER ROOT

2 TABLESPOONS LOW-SODIUM SOY SAUCE

Make the filling: Steep the tea in ½ cup boiling water for 5 minutes and drain. (See page 10 for ways to use the liquid.) Mince the tea leaves. Combine tea leaves with remaining filling ingredients in a large bowl.

Set up a space for folding the dumplings. Place a bowl of cold water, the wrappers and the filling around your work area. Cover the wrappers with a damp paper towel to prevent drying. Dip one edge of a wrapper into the water. Spoon about 1½ teaspoons of filling onto the center of the wrapper. Fold the wrapper over to form a half circle, pressing the dry edge to the wet edge. Pinch the edges together to seal the dumpling. Place dumplings on a floured plate and loosely cover with a towel to keep them from drying. Repeat with remaining filling and wrappers.

Mix 1 tablespoon of the oil with ¼ cup of the water in a large nonstick skillet. Place half of the dumplings in a spiraling circle in the skillet, leaving just a little space between them.

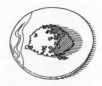

1. Dip one edge of the wrapper in water. Place a heaping teaspoon of filling in the center.

2. Fold the wrapper in half to form a half circle.

3. Pinch the edges together to seal.

Cover and cook over medium heat until dumplings puff up and are light brown on the bottom and the liquid evaporates, 8 to 10 minutes. Repeat with remaining dumplings, oil and water.

Garnish with green onion and edible flowers, if using, and serve hot with the Chile-Garlic Oil.

Makes 35 to 40 dumplings

VARIATION

IF YOU USE THE GYOZA PACK, DIP ONE EDGE OF A WRAPPER INTO THE WATER. PLACE THE WRAPPER IN THE GYOZA PACK. PLACE 1 HEAPING TEASPOON OF FILLING IN THE CENTER OF THE WRAPPER AND CLOSE THE PACK TIGHTLY.

DIM SUM

LITERALLY "HEART'S DELIGHT," DIM SUM WERE FIRST PRE-
PARED SEVEN CENTURIES AGO IN THE COURT OF THE SUNG
DYNASTY. LATER THESE SUCCULENT, BITE-SIZE DELICACIES
SPREAD TO TEAHOUSES ALL OVER CHINA. THESE TASTE
TREATS ARE MADE WITH A WIDE RANGE OF FILLINGS, AND ARE
STEAMED, BAKED, ROASTED, PAN-FRIED AND DEEP-FRIED. IN
SOUTHERN CHINA, PEOPLE DEVELOPED A UNIQUE PASSION
FOR DIM SUM AND TEA. THEY INVENTED TWO THOUSAND
VARIETIES OF THESE TEATIME SNACKS. YOUNG AND OLD,
MALE AND FEMALE, ALL ENJOY DRINKING TEA AND SAMPLING
DELICIOUS DIM SUM. FRIENDS AND FAMILY GATHERING
TOGETHER AT A RESTAURANT, DRINKING TEA AND SAMPLING
DIM SUM BECAME THE MOST IMPORTANT SOCIAL EVENT IN
SOUTHERN CHINA. MANY BUSINESS NEGOTIATIONS BEGIN AT
THIS TIME AND FINISH AT THE OFFICE.

TODAY, YOU CAN FIND SOME CHINESE RESTAURANTS
SERVING DIM SUM IN THIS COUNTRY, ESPECIALLY RESTAU-
RANTS IN CHINATOWNS. REMEMBER, DON'T FEAST ON JUST
ONE OR TWO ITEMS, SAMPLE THEM ALL. DRINK TEA BETWEEN
SERVINGS OF DIFFERENT TYPES OF DIM SUM, SO THE TASTE
OF ONE DOES NOT MAR THAT OF ANOTHER.

Succulent Seafood, Chicken and Meat

Chinese believe that yin and yang are two opposing forces that are mutually dependent. Yin is passive, cool, dark and associated with femininity. Yang is active, hot, bright and associated with masculinity. To put it another way, yin represents the dark side of a mountain while yang represents the sunny side. Yin symbolizes night, yang symbolizes day; yin represents winter, yang summer; yin represents mild, light food, yang hot, rich food.

Chinese physicians view a healthy diet as one in which both yin and yang are in harmony. Yin foods soothe and moisturize the body. They are soft and cool, for example, green tea, green leafy vegetables, plain steamed rice and cold drinks. Yin cooking methods are steaming and simmering. Yang foods are hot, dry and spicy, for example, red meat, chilies, garlic and ginger. They increase perspiration. Yang cooking methods are deep-frying or stir-frying without sauce, or smoking.

It is simple to create a harmony of yin and yang within an individual dish or within a meal, such as Emperor's Shrimp, which is shrimp marinated in Spicy Sesame Sauce (yang) balanced by bell peppers and tea (yin). In Green Tea- and Orange-Smoked Salmon, cooking with smoke (yang) is balanced by the tea, raw rice and lettuce leaves (yin). Meatballs with Spicy Coconut Sauce (yang) is best served with plain steamed rice or Spinach Salad with Avocado and Tofu (page 121), which is yin, to balance the heat and spice.

Cooking with green tea is a simple and healthy way to achieve harmony and balance in your diet.

Orange-Flavored Scallops

Don't be puzzled if you go to a Chinese home and see orange peel laid out to dry. It's not that someone forgot to throw them away; the family is simply following the Chinese practice of food as medicine. Oranges and orange peel, fresh or dried, are commonly used in Chinese cooking because orange peel is believed to clear the lungs and sooth an irritated throat. Their sweet-and-sour flavors go well with fresh seafood.

2 ORANGES

1 POUND SEA SCALLOPS

2 TABLESPOONS RICE WINE

1 TABLESPOON MINCED GINGER ROOT

4 TEASPOONS CORNSTARCH

4 TABLESPOONS CANOLA OIL

1 TABLESPOON LOOSE GREEN TEA

3 TABLESPOONS 2-INCH-LONG MATCHSTICK-SIZE
GINGER ROOT STRIPS

2 CLOVES GARLIC, MINCED

2 SMALL LEEKS, WHITE PARTS ONLY, CUT INTO
3-INCH-LONG MATCHSTICK-SIZE STRIPS

4 MEDIUM CARROTS, PEELED, CUT INTO
3-INCH-LONG MATCHSTICK-SIZE STRIPS

2 TABLESPOONS BREWED GREEN TEA (PAGE 7)

2 TABLESPOONS LIME JUICE

SALT AND WHITE PEPPER, TO TASTE

2 TABLESPOONS FRESH CILANTRO LEAVES

Remove just the orange-colored zest from the oranges. Cut into matchstick-size 1-inch-long pieces; set 3 tablespoons aside. Juice the oranges, reserving ½ cup.

In a medium bowl, combine the scallops, orange juice, wine, minced ginger and cornstarch. Cover and marinate the scallops for 20 minutes in the refrigerator.

Drain the marinade from the scallops. Heat 3 tablespoons of the oil in a nonstick wok or cooking pan over high heat and swirl to coat pan. Add the tea leaves, ginger pieces, garlic and orange peel and sauté until fragrant, about 30 seconds. Add the scallops and stir-fry until scallops are crisp on the outsides, about 2 minutes. Transfer the scallops to a bowl. Set aside.

Heat the remaining 1 tablespoon oil in the wok over medium-high heat. Add the leeks and carrots and stir-fry until leeks soften, 1 to 2 minutes. Add the brewed tea and lime juice. Return the scallops to the pan and stir-fry until heated through. Season with salt and pepper. Garnish with cilantro leaves and serve hot.

Makes 4 to 6 servings

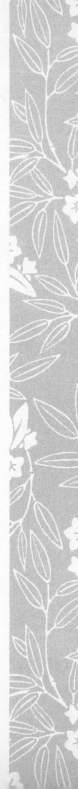

Steamed Scallops and Tofu with Ginger

Tofu, scallops, green tea and steam cooking methods are yin elements in Chinese medicine. The yang elements of ginger and a spicy sauce make this dish well balanced on its own.

8 LARGE SEA SCALLOPS

3 TABLESPOONS GINGER AND GARLIC SAUCE (PAGE 43)

2 TEASPOONS LOOSE GREEN TEA

1 (12-OZ.) PACKAGE FIRM SILKEN TOFU

8 THIN SLICES GINGER ROOT

2 GREEN ONIONS, WHITE PART ONLY, CUT INTO 2-INCH-LONG MATCHSTICK-SIZE STRIPS

SPICY LEMON-BASIL SAUCE (PAGE 47), TO SERVE

Add the scallops and Ginger and Garlic Sauce to a bowl and stir to coat. Cover and marinate the scallops for 20 minutes in the refrigerator.

Soak the tea leaves in ½ cup boiling water about 5 minutes. Drain and reserve the tea leaves. (See page 10 for ways to use the liquid.)

Cut the tofu in half horizontally to make 2 sheets. Cut each half into quarters to make a total of 8 rectangles.

Place tofu in a heatproof dish. Top each piece with a scallop. Layer the ginger, green onions and ½ teaspoon tea leaves on each scallop. Spoon remaining marinade sauce over all.

In a large pot, bring about 4 cups water to a boil. Place the dish in a steamer rack over the boiling water. Cover and steam over high heat until scallops turn opaque, 5 to 6 minutes. Carefully discard steaming liquid. Serve hot with Spicy Lemon-Basil Sauce.

Makes 8 servings

Mussels in Lemon Grass– Green Tea Wine Sauce

Fresh mussels taste sweet and delicate. When you buy them, they should be alive. The way to tell is to tap the mussels gently. They should close their shells quickly. If you want to make sure the mussels are absolutely clean, soak them in clean cold water for about 2 hours, changing the water twice. I like to throw in a couple of tea bags. The mussels will release any grit and inhale the flavor of the tea.

Serve with steamed rice and vegetables as a main dish or as an appetizer.

1 POUND FRESH MUSSELS IN SHELLS

1 TABLESPOON CANOLA OIL

4 CLOVES GARLIC, MINCED

½ TABLESPOON MINCED GINGER ROOT

2 STEMS LEMON GRASS, BOTTOMS ONLY, CHOPPED

½ FRESH RED CHILE PEPPER (OPTIONAL)

4 FRESH CILANTRO SPRIGS

SAUCE

½ CUP BREWED GREEN TEA (PAGE 7)

2 TABLESPOONS RICE WINE

1 TABLESPOON FISH SAUCE

1 TABLESPOON LIME JUICE

Before cooking, tap any open mussels with a spoon and discard any that don't close. Scrub the outside of the mussels with a brush. Remove the beards by pulling, and discard.

Make the sauce: Combine all ingredients in a small bowl.

Heat the oil in a nonstick wok or cooking pan over medium-high heat and swirl to coat pan. Add the garlic, ginger, lemon grass and chile, if using. Stir-fry until fragrant, about 10 seconds. Reduce heat to medium. Add the mussels and cook for 3 minutes.

Add the sauce and toss mussels to combine. Cover the wok. Cook, stirring occasionally, until mussels open, about 2 minutes. (Do not overcook, or mussels will become tough.)

Discard any mussels that have not opened. Garnish with cilantro. Serve hot.

Makes 4 servings

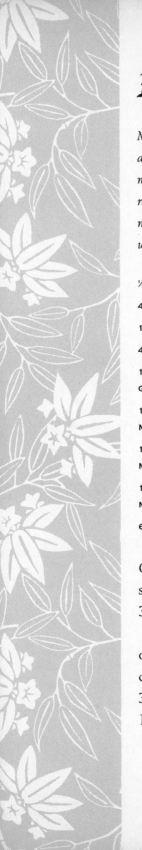

Emperor's Shrimp

Most of the shrimp sold in the store has been flash-frozen. I always keep some in my freezer. They are ideal for last-minute meals. Even better, shrimp, like other shellfish, are low in saturated fat. If shrimp is pink, it has been cooked and has lost much of its flavor. Look for grayish raw shrimp. Serve this dish with noodles or steamed rice.

¼ CUP SPICY SESAME SAUCE (PAGE 42)

4 TEASPOONS CORNSTARCH

1 POUND MEDIUM RAW SHRIMP, SHELLED AND DEVEINED

4 TABLESPOONS CANOLA OIL

1 TABLESPOON LOOSE GREEN TEA, PREFERABLY GUNPOWDER

1 MEDIUM GREEN BELL PEPPER, CUT INTO 2-INCH-LONG MATCHSTICK-SIZE STRIPS

1 MEDIUM RED BELL PEPPER, CUT INTO 2-INCH-LONG MATCHSTICK-SIZE STRIPS

1 MEDIUM WHITE ONION, CUT INTO 2-INCH-LONG MATCHSTICK-SIZE STRIPS

6 TABLESPOONS CASHEW NUTS, TOASTED (PAGE 124)

Combine sauce and cornstarch in a bowl. Add shrimp and toss to coat. Cover and refrigerate for 30 minutes.

Heat 2 tablespoons of the oil in a nonstick wok or cooking pan over medium-high heat and swirl to coat pan. Add the tea and sauté until fragrant, about 30 seconds. Add the shrimp and stir-fry until pink, 1 to 2 minutes. Remove and place in a bowl.

Heat the remaining 2 tablespoons oil in the wok. Add the bell peppers and onion and stir-fry until peppers soften, 1 to 2 minutes. Return the shrimp to the wok and stir-fry until heated through. Stir in cashew nuts. Serve hot.

Makes 4 servings

Green-Tea-and-Orange-Smoked Salmon

Oily fish such as salmon contain omega-3 fatty acids, which can protect against heart disease, help maintain vision by protecting the retina and help brains cells transmit electrical signals. Because our bodies don't produce omega-3 fatty acids, we must obtain them from foods or supplements. Other foods containing omega-3 fatty acids are leafy vegetables, canola oil and nuts. Give your body a nice boost with this dish.

Smoking the salmon over green tea, raw rice and orange peel gives this dish a wonderful flavor. It is also a low-fat way to cook salmon.

2 POUNDS SKINLESS SALMON FILLETS

½ CUP GREEN TEA–GINGER SAUCE (PAGE 49)

½ CUP THAI SAUCE (PAGE 50), FOR SERVING (OPTIONAL)

FOR SMOKING

3 LARGE LETTUCE LEAVES

⅓ CUP LOOSE GREEN TEA OR CONTENTS OF 6 TEA BAGS

½ CUP RAW RICE

2 TABLESPOONS SUGAR

½ CUP CHOPPED FRESH ORANGE OR LEMON PEEL

Cut 1-inch-deep diagonal slashes about 2 inches apart on one side of the salmon fillets. Place the fillets, slashed side down, in a large bowl with the

Green Tea–Ginger Sauce. Cover and refrigerate for at least 30 minutes, or overnight for the best flavor.

Line the bottom of an old large pan with foil and line the foil with lettuce leaves. Add the green tea, rice, sugar and orange peel, mixing them together on the lettuce.

Place a steamer rack in the pan and place the salmon fillets on it. Tightly cover the pan with foil and a lid (see page 18). Cook over medium heat for 25 to 30 minutes (depending on the thickness of the fillets), until salmon browns and easily flakes with a fork. Remove from heat before opening. Serve hot, with Thai Sauce if desired.

Makes 6 servings

Green Tea Steamed Sea Bass

Growing up next to the Yangtze River, I always had a passion for fresh fish. In the summer and fall I like to go fishing to catch my own fish. When choosing fresh whole fish at the market, look for ones with clear eyes and shiny skin.

Serve this fish with steamed rice.

1 (1½-LB.) FRESH WHOLE SEA BASS OR TROUT, WITHOUT HEAD

2 TABLESPOONS FINELY CHOPPED GINGER ROOT

4 CLOVES GARLIC, MINCED

2 TEASPOONS SESAME OIL

2 TABLESPOONS BROWN RICE WINE

2 TABLESPOONS LOW-SODIUM SOY SAUCE

2 TABLESPOONS LEMON JUICE

SALT AND WHITE PEPPER, TO TASTE

4 BAGS GREEN TEA

2 SMALL LEEKS, WHITE PART ONLY, CUT INTO 2-INCH-LONG MATCHSTICK-SIZE STRIPS

Cut 3 or 4 (¼-inch-deep) diagonal slashes along both sides of the fish. Dry the outside of the fish with a paper towel. Place on a heatproof plate.

Mix the ginger, garlic, sesame oil, rice wine, soy sauce, lemon juice, salt and pepper in a small bowl. Spoon the mixture into the body cavity and outside of the fish. Cover and refrigerate 40 minutes.

Bring 4 cups of water to a boil in a steamer pot. Add the tea bags. Cover the fish with the leeks. Place the plate on a steamer rack in pot. Cover and steam over high heat until the thickest part of the fish flakes easily with a fork, 10 to 15 minutes.

Makes 4 servings

Grilled Fish in Grape Leaves

One summer evening while I was sitting under the grape arbor in front of my house, I remembered a dish I had eaten in the Philippines called fish in banana leaf. Because banana leaves are scarce in Colorado, I decided to replace the banana leaves with my big green grape leaves. I gave the recipe to my neighbors and friends, and since then my grape leaves never go to waste. You can also steam the fish; see the variation.

⅓ CUP SPICY SESAME SAUCE (PAGE 42)

4 WHITE FISH FILLETS, ABOUT 1½ POUNDS

20 LARGE GRAPE LEAVES

TOPPING

4 TEASPOONS LOOSE GREEN TEA

3 TABLESPOONS THINLY SHREDDED GINGER ROOT

4 GREEN ONIONS, THINLY SHREDDED

½ CUP OYSTER MUSHROOM, MINCED

2 FRESH RED CHILE PEPPERS, SEEDED AND MINCED

2 TEASPOONS SESAME OIL

Pour the sauce over the fish in a large bowl. Cover and refrigerate for 30 minutes.

In a big pot, bring 5 cups water to a boil. Dip grape leaves into the boiling water for about 2 seconds to soften. Drip dry.

Preheat a grill. Make the topping: Soak the tea leaves in ½ cup boiling water about 5 minutes. Drain and mince the tea leaves. (See page 10 for ways to use the liquid.) Combine all the ingredients except sesame oil in a small bowl.

Center 4 or 5 grape leaves on a large piece of foil. Place on them one of the fish fillets. Place one-fourth of the topping and ½ teaspoon sesame oil on top of the fish. Fold leaves over fish, then fold foil around fish to enclose it. Repeat with remaining fish and topping.

Grill the fish, turning once, until the fish flakes easily, 7 to 10 minutes.

Place the fish on a serving platter. Open foil and grape leaves. Serve hot.

Makes 4 servings

VARIATION

TO STEAM: PLACE 4 TEA BAGS IN THE BOILING WATER USED FOR SOFTENING GRAPE LEAVES. PLACE WRAPPED FISH ON A STEAM RACK OVER BOILING TEA OVER HIGH HEAT. STEAM UNTIL FISH FLAKES WITH A FORK, 8 TO 10 MINUTES.

Stuffed Crispy Whole Trout

Aren't you always impressed when people serve you a whole fish? Now you can impress your guests. Even better, chances are they never had a whole fish cooked with green tea. Grilling the fish instead of pan-frying will save you cleanup time in the kitchen and cut down on the fat. You can also broil the fish.

2 (1-LB.) WHOLE TROUT, CLEANED AND SCALED, WITHOUT HEADS

SALT AND BLACK PEPPER, TO TASTE

1 TABLESPOON LOOSE GREEN TEA

3 TABLESPOONS FINELY SHREDDED GINGER ROOT

3 GREEN ONIONS (GREEN AND WHITE PARTS), FINELY SHREDDED

3 FRESH CILANTRO SPRIGS, CUT INTO 2-INCH-LONG PIECES

1½ FRESH RED CHILE PEPPERS, FINELY SHREDDED

2 TABLESPOONS CANOLA OIL

1 SMALL YELLOW BELL PEPPER, CUT INTO 2-INCH SQUARES

1 SMALL RED BELL PEPPER, CUT INTO 2-INCH SQUARES

½ CUP THAI SAUCE (PAGE 50)

Cut 3 or 4 (¼-inch-deep) diagonal slashes along both sides of each fish. Dry the outsides of the fish with a paper towel. Rub the salt and pepper into the slashes and inside each fish.

Soak the tea leaves in ½ cup boiling water about 5 minutes. Drain and reserve the tea leaves. (See page 10 for ways of using the liquid.) Stuff half of the ginger, green onions, tea leaves, cilantro and chile peppers into slashes and inside each fish.

Heat the oil in a nonstick stovetop grill over medium-high heat and swirl to coat surface. Place both fish on grill and partially cover. Grill the fish until the skin is crisp and brown, about 8 minutes. Turn the fish and place the bell peppers around them. Grill fish until crispy and bell peppers are light golden and tender. Transfer to a serving plate. Arrange bell peppers around or on top of the fish.

Bring the sauce to a boil in a small saucepan. Pour sauce over the fish and bell peppers. Serve hot.

Makes 4 servings

VARIATION

TO BROIL THE FISH, PREHEAT BROILER. BRUSH EACH SIDE OF THE FISH WITH CANOLA OIL. SET THE FISH IN A NONSTICK BAKING PAN THAT HAS BEEN LIGHTLY COATED WITH COOKING SPRAY. BROIL THE FISH ON THE MIDDLE RACK UNTIL THE SKIN CRISPS AND BROWNS, 10 TO 13 MINUTES PER SIDE, TURNING ONCE AND ADDING THE BELL PEPPERS.

Grilled Teriyaki Chicken

Chicken breasts are low in fat and easy to prepare. They also freeze well. I like to use natural meat and chicken that are hormone and antibiotic free. Some chickens are even raised on a vegetarian diet. Natural meat is available at health food stores and some supermarkets.

Teriyaki Chicken goes well with vegetables and rice.

4 SKINLESS, BONELESS CHICKEN BREAST HALVES

MARINADE

1 TABLESPOON FISH SAUCE

1 TABLESPOON RICE VINEGAR

⅛ TEASPOON WHITE PEPPER

4 TEASPOONS CORNSTARCH

1 TABLESPOON MINCED GARLIC

1 TABLESPOON MINCED FRESH ORANGE ZEST

2 GREEN ONIONS (GREEN AND WHITE PARTS), MINCED

SAUCE

½ CUP BREWED GREEN TEA (PAGE 7)

1 TEASPOON HONEY

1 TEASPOON LEMON JUICE

Make the marinade: Mix the fish sauce, vinegar and pepper in a medium bowl. Dissolve the cornstarch in the vinegar mixture. Stir in the garlic, orange zest and green onions. Toss the chicken with the marinade. Cover and refrigerate for 2 hours.

Remove the chicken from the marinade, reserving marinade. Preheat a grill. Place chicken on grill and cook for 8 to 10 minutes. Turn and brush with reserved marinade. Grill 8 to 10 minutes, or until tender and no longer pink in centers.

Make the sauce: Combine all sauce ingredients in a small bowl. Serve as a dipping sauce with the chicken.

Makes 4 servings

Spicy and Colorful Chicken Salad

Serve this delicious salad with fresh garlic bread. It makes a simple, nutritious meal for a hot summer night or weekend picnic.

4 SKINLESS, BONELESS CHICKEN BREAST HALVES

⅔ CUP SPICY CILANTRO SAUCE (PAGE 44)

4 CUPS CURLY ENDIVE OR 1 (4-OZ.) BAG BABY GREEN SALAD MIX

½ RED BELL PEPPER, CUT INTO THIN STRIPS

½ YELLOW BELL PEPPER, CUT INTO THIN STRIPS

1 SMALL RED ONION, THINLY SLICED

1 JALAPEÑO OR SERRANO CHILE PEPPER, SEEDED AND FINELY MINCED (FOR A HOTTER SALAD, KEEP THE SEEDS IN)

½ CUP HONEY-GINGER SAUCE (PAGE 46)

2 TABLESPOONS PINE NUTS, TOASTED (SEE TIP, PAGE 124)

Toss chicken with the Spicy Cilantro Sauce. Cover and refrigerate for 1 hour or overnight.

Remove the chicken from the marinade, reserving marinade. Preheat a grill. Place chicken on grill and cook for 8 to 10 minutes on each side or until tender and no longer pink, turning and brushing with the remaining marinade halfway through grilling.

Combine the endive, bell peppers, onion and chile in a large bowl. Add the Honey-Ginger Sauce and toss to mix. Arrange greens mixture on 4 plates. Top with chicken and pine nuts.

Makes 4 servings

VARIATIONS

TO BAKE CHICKEN: PREHEAT OVEN TO 400F (205C). PLACE CHICKEN ON A LIGHTLY OILED BAKING SHEET. BAKE 20 TO 25 MINUTES, UNTIL NO PINK REMAINS IN CENTERS.

IF YOU ARE IN A HURRY AND WANT A SIMPLER VERSION, STOP BY YOUR NATURAL FOODS STORE DELI AND BUY A ROASTED CHICKEN AND A BAG OF SALAD. IN NO TIME YOU WILL BE ENJOYING A HEALTHFUL AND SATISFYING MEAL.

Lemon and Ginger Pork with Vegetables

By using frozen vegetables and precut meat, you can enjoy this delicious dish without much effort. You can even marinate the meat the night before. The Honey-Ginger Sauce will give the dish extra flavor, but if you are pressed for time, season the dish with salt and pepper according to your taste.

Serve over noodles or rice.

2 TABLESPOONS SOY SAUCE

1 TABLESPOON LEMON JUICE

1 TEASPOON CORNSTARCH

1 POUND PORK TENDERLOIN, CUT INTO LONG MATCHSTICK-SIZE STRIPS

2 TABLESPOONS CHILE-GARLIC OIL (PAGE 45)

½ TABLESPOON LOOSE GREEN TEA

1 TABLESPOON MINCED GINGER ROOT

3 TABLESPOONS FRESHLY GRATED LEMON PEEL

1 (16-OZ.) PACKAGE MIXED FROZEN VEGETABLES, WITH BROCCOLI, CARROTS AND WATER CHESTNUTS

¼ CUP HONEY-GINGER SAUCE (PAGE 46), OPTIONAL

SALT AND BLACK PEPPER, TO TASTE

Combine the soy sauce, lemon juice and cornstarch in a medium bowl. Add the pork and toss to combine. Cover and refrigerate for 30 minutes or longer.

Arrange the rest of the ingredients near the cooking area.

Heat the oil in a nonstick wok or cooking pan over medium-high heat and swirl to coat pan. Add the tea, ginger and lemon peel and stir-fry until fragrant, about 30 seconds. Add the pork and stir-fry until no pink remains, about 2 minutes.

Add the vegetables and stir-fry 2 minutes. Stir in Honey-Ginger Sauce, if using. Reduce the heat and stir-fry until vegetables are crisp, tender and heated through, 3 to 5 minutes. Season with salt and pepper.

Makes 4 servings

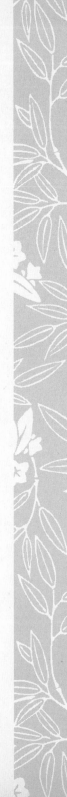

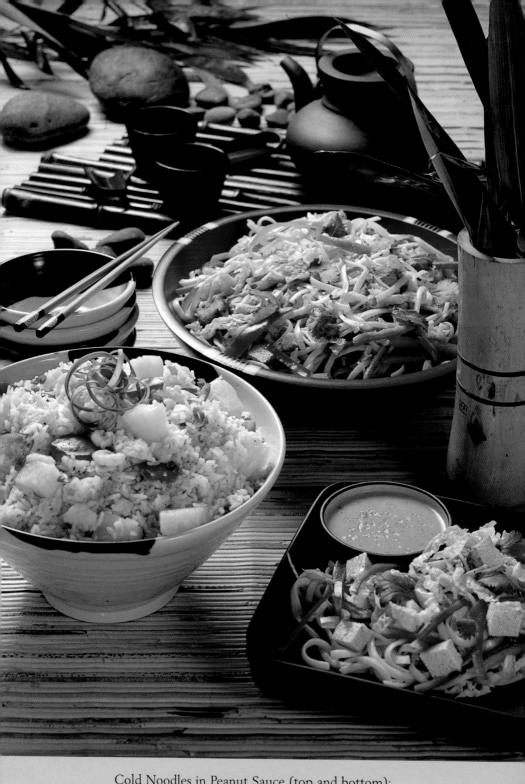

Cold Noodles in Peanut Sauce (top and bottom);
Colorful Fried Rice (left).

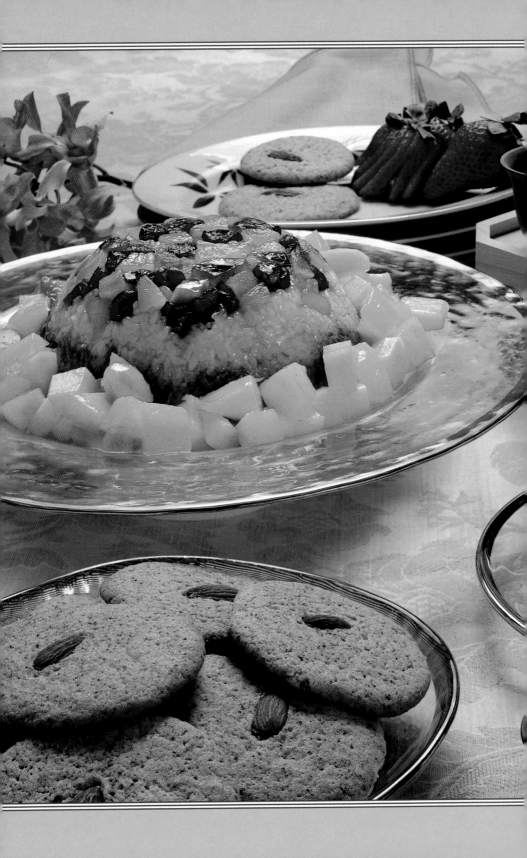

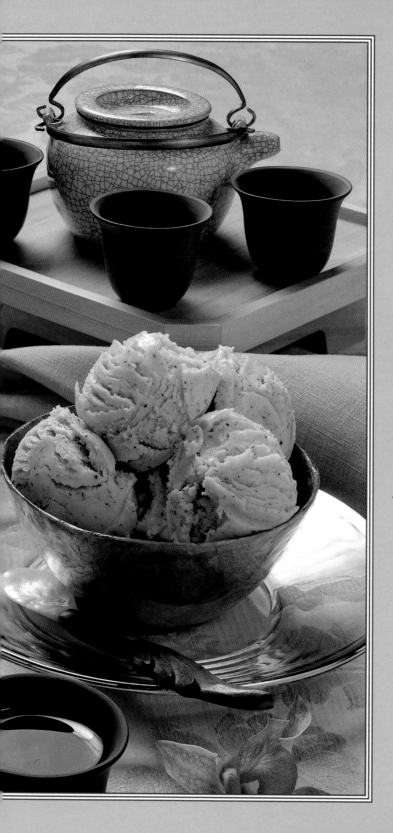

CLOCKWISE
FROM TOP
LEFT:
Sweet
Eight-Treasure
Rice Pudding;
Green Tea
Ice Cream;
Jasmine Almond
Cookies.

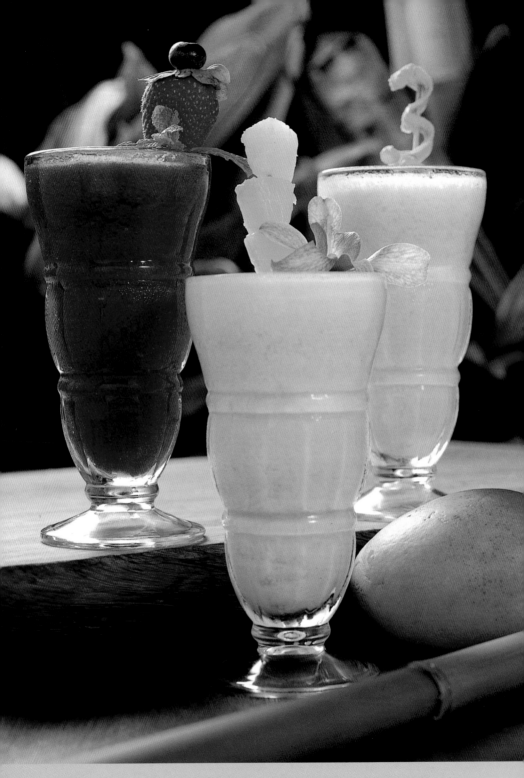

Three-Berry Shake (top left); Green Tea, Mango and Yogurt Smoothie
(top right); New Age Piña Colada (bottom).

Spicy Beef with Carrots and Leeks

Enjoy this dish the way a Chinese person would. The fresh vegetables should be the focus of this dish, while the meat is only for flavoring. Use precut stir-fry beef and bagged shredded carrots or even frozen vegetables if you're in a hurry. Serve with rice or noodles.

1 POUND BEEF EYE OF ROUND, CUT INTO ¼-INCH-WIDE STRIPS

2 TABLESPOONS CHILE-GARLIC OIL (PAGE 45)

1 TABLESPOON LOOSE GREEN TEA

6 SMALL DRIED RED CHILE PEPPERS

1 LARGE CARROT, CUT INTO 2-INCH-LONG MATCHSTICK-SIZE STRIPS

2 SMALL LEEKS, WHITE PART ONLY, CUT INTO 2-INCH-LONG MATCHSTICK-SIZE STRIPS

2 SMALL FRESH GREEN CHILE PEPPERS, THINLY SLICED

⅓ CUP GINGER AND GARLIC SAUCE (PAGE 43)

SALT AND BLACK PEPPER, TO TASTE

½ CUP CHOPPED ROASTED PEANUTS

MARINADE

1 TABLESPOON SOY SAUCE

2 TEASPOONS RICE WINE

1 TABLESPOON MINCED GARLIC

1 TABLESPOON MINCED GINGER ROOT

1 TEASPOON CORNSTARCH

Make the marinade: Mix all the marinade ingredients in a bowl. Add the beef and toss to coat. Cover and refrigerate for 30 minutes or longer.

Arrange the marinade and other ingredients in the cooking area. Heat the oil in a large nonstick wok or cooking pan over medium-high heat and swirl to coat pan. Add the green tea and dried chile peppers and stir-fry until fragrant, about 30 seconds. Add the beef mixture and stir-fry until no pink remains, about 2 minutes.

Add the carrot, leeks and chile peppers and stir-fry for 2 minutes. Stir in the ginger-garlic sauce, reduce the heat and cook for 2 minutes. Season with salt and pepper.

Transfer to a serving bowl and garnish with the peanuts.

Makes 4 servings

Meatballs in Spicy Coconut Sauce

These meatballs are perfect for any occasion. Make them ahead of time, and keep them chilled or frozen until you are ready to cook them.

You must plan ahead when making this recipe to allow for the tofu to be frozen. I have found that freezing the tofu first and then thawing it not only helps remove excess water but gives the tofu a firmer, spongier, chewier texture. Serve over steamed rice or noodles.

2 TEASPOONS LOOSE GREEN TEA

8 OUNCES (½ PACKAGE) FRESH EXTRA FIRM TOFU, FROZEN AND THEN THAWED IN HOT WATER

¼ POUND LEAN GROUND PORK OR GROUND BEEF

1 EGG, LIGHTLY BEATEN

1 TABLESPOON CORNSTARCH

½ TABLESPOON GRATED LEMON PEEL

1 TEASPOON SESAME OIL

2 TEASPOONS MINCED GINGER ROOT

5 SPRIGS CILANTRO, MINCED

1 FRESH GREEN OR RED CHILE PEPPER, FINELY CHOPPED

1 TABLESPOON CANOLA OIL

2 TEASPOONS FISH SAUCE, OR TO TASTE

SPICY COCONUT SAUCE

½ CUP UNSWEETENED LIGHT COCONUT MILK

1 TABLESPOON COCONUT FLAVORED YOGURT

5 SPRIGS CILANTRO, CHOPPED

1 FRESH RED CHILE PEPPER, CHOPPED

1 TABLESPOON FRESHLY GRATED LEMON PEEL

Soak the tea leaves in ½ cup boiling water about 3 minutes. Drain, reserving liquid for the sauce, and mince the tea leaves. Set aside.

Make the sauce: Mix all the sauce ingredients, including the reserved liquid tea, in a bowl and set aside.

Place the tofu on a cutting board. Press out the excess liquid with a plate. Mash the tofu in a large bowl. Add the tea leaves, pork, egg, cornstarch, lemon peel, sesame oil, ginger, cilantro and chile and mix well. Divide the mixture into 15 equal portions, about 2 tablespoons each. Roll each portion into a ball.

Heat the oil in a wide nonstick frying pan over medium-high heat. Add the meatballs, and fry, turning occasionally, until browned on all sides, 7 to 10 minutes.

Add the coconut sauce. Cover and simmer for 8 to 10 minutes. Season with the fish sauce. Serve hot.

Makes 15 meatballs

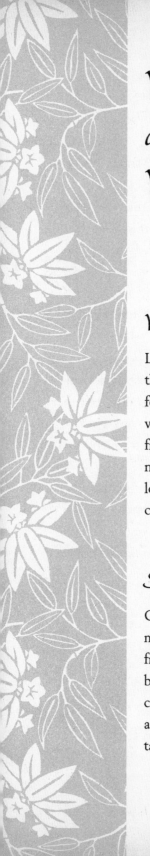

Venerable Soy and Vibrant Vegetables

Vegetables

Last year I took a trip to Russia. For ten days I went through vegetable withdrawal, because there were so few available. One night I even dreamed of planting vegetables outside my hotel. Vegetables, fresh or frozen, provide your body with valuable vitamins, minerals and antioxidants. They are high in fiber and low in fat. Vegetables help with your digestion and cleanse your body.

Soy

Growing up in China, I enjoyed soymilk as a regular, nutritious part of my diet. My grandmother served fresh tofu and vegetables at almost every meal. Soy-based foods filled my empty stomach, satisfied my craving for sweets, comforted me when I was sick, and cheered me when I was sad. Most of all they taught me respect for natural foods.

For centuries much of Asia has favored high-protein tofu, a vegetarian food made from soybeans. Even today, tofu and other soy products are the primary source of protein in the daily diet of many Chinese.

Tofu is high in calcium, potassium and vitamins B and E. It is low in sodium and fat and is cholesterol-free.

The average American would be surprised by the many varieties of tofu available on the market. For fresh tofu, I prefer low-fat silken Mori Nu, which is sold in about 12-ounce aseptic (shelf-stable) cartons. With only 1 gram of fat per serving, it is ideal for soups, desserts and dressings. It can be stored on the shelves for months. It is great for last-minute dinner ideas. Another brand I like is White Wave, which comes in regular and flavored varieties.

Soybean cake, or baked tofu, is fresh tofu that has been pressed to remove the moisture, then cooked in flavored water or baked, then marinated in sauce. There are many different brands available on the market, many with surprisingly complex and meaty flavors. I use them to flavor a dish. It's ideal for stir-frying. Try to find a brand that is low in sodium.

Ever wonder why soy can do so much good for our bodies? Research suggests that the active ingredients in soy protein are antioxidants called isoflavones, which have been shown to reduce the risk of cancer, heart disease and osteoporosis. Soy protein also contains plant-based estrogens, which may ease the symptoms of menopause without increasing the risk of cancer.

Spinach Salad with Avocado and Tofu

The sharp taste of the parsley in this salad is a perfect complement to sweet ripe avocados and chilled tofu. Served with fresh bread, this tasty and beautiful salad makes a great lunch.

1 (12-OZ.) PACKAGE REDUCED-FAT EXTRA FIRM SILKEN TOFU, DRAINED AND CUT INTO ½-INCH CUBES

3 TABLESPOONS HONEY-GINGER SAUCE (PAGE 46)

2 CUPS BABY SPINACH LEAVES, LARGE STEMS REMOVED

½ CUP TIGHTLY PACKED PARSLEY LEAVES, CHOPPED

1 AVOCADO, PEELED, PITTED AND CUBED

¼ CUP PINE NUTS, TOASTED (PAGE 124)

SPICY GARLIC DRESSING

½ FRESH RED CHILE PEPPER, MINCED

1 TABLESPOON MINCED LEMON PEEL

2 CLOVES GARLIC, FINELY MINCED

2 TABLESPOONS LOOSE GREEN TEA

2 TABLESPOONS EXTRA-VIRGIN OLIVE OIL

½ TABLESPOON RED VINEGAR

1 TABLESPOON LEMON JUICE

⅛ TEASPOON SALT

¼ TEASPOON BLACK PEPPER

In a medium bowl, marinate the tofu in the sauce in the refrigerator for 1 hour.

Make the dressing: In a small bowl, combine all the dressing ingredients. Mix thoroughly.

In a large bowl, combine the spinach and parsley. Arrange on 4 to 6 plates. Sprinkle with the tofu and avocado. Drizzle with the dressing and garnish with the pine nuts.

Makes 4 to 6 servings

TIP

YOU CAN MARINATE THE TOFU AND MAKE THE SALAD DRESS-ING AHEAD OF TIME. BUT FOR THE BEST COLOR AND TASTE, CUT THE AVOCADO AND ASSEMBLE THE DISH JUST BEFORE SERVING.

Garden Salad with Marble Eggs

This delicious and colorful salad will do more than tantalize your taste buds. It will provide your body with a burst of important vitamins and minerals.

Eggs are an important source of protein in the Asian diet. They are included in many dishes.

3 MARBLE EGGS (PAGE 85)

1 MEDIUM CARROT

1 GREEN ONION

1 (ABOUT 4-OZ.) BAG BABY GREEN SALAD MIX

½ RED BELL PEPPER, CUT INTO MATCHSTICK-SIZE STRIPS

½ YELLOW BELL PEPPER, CUT INTO MATCHSTICK-SIZE STRIPS

2 TABLESPOONS PINE NUTS, TOASTED (SEE TIP)

DRESSING

4 OUNCES (½ CUP) REDUCED-FAT SOFT SILKEN TOFU

1 TABLESPOON LEMON JUICE

½ CUP BREWED GREEN TEA (PAGE 7)

½ CUP PLAIN SOY MILK

1 TABLESPOON RICE VINEGAR

1 TEASPOON MINCED GINGER ROOT

2 CLOVES GARLIC, MINCED

2 TEASPOONS SESAME OIL

SALT AND BLACK PEPPER, TO TASTE

Drain and peel the eggs. Cut each egg lengthwise into quarters. Set aside.

Wash and peel the carrots. Cut diagonally into thin slices, then cut lengthwise into matchstick-size strips. Cut green onion into 2-inch diagonals, then cut lengthwise into matchstick-size pieces. Toss together the salad mix, bell peppers and carrot and onion in a large serving bowl.

Make the dressing: Combine all dressing ingredients except salt and black pepper in a blender. Puree until smooth and creamy. Season with salt and pepper.

Pour dressing over salad and toss again. Top with eggs and pine nuts.

Makes 4 servings

TIP

TO TOAST PINE NUTS OR OTHER NUTS: PREHEAT OVEN TO 350F (175C). SPREAD PINE NUTS IN A BAKING SHEET IN A SINGLE LAYER. BAKE 9 TO 10 MINUTES, UNTIL NUTS TURN CRISP AND GOLDEN, STIRRING OCCASIONALLY.

Roasted Peppers and Potato Salad

Roasting the bell peppers changes their texture and enhances their flavor, adding a rich sweetness. You'll be amazed that anything this low in fat can taste so great.

3 BELL PEPPERS, 1 RED, 1 YELLOW AND 1 GREEN

2 BAGS GREEN TEA

1 LARGE (ABOUT 8-OZ.) RED POTATO

¼ CUP THAI SAUCE (PAGE 50) OR HONEY-GINGER
SAUCE (PAGE 46)

1 GREEN ONION (GREEN PART ONLY), CHOPPED

Preheat the grill or broiler. Grill bell peppers on all sides until they are completely blistered and charred, about 8 minutes.

Transfer the bell peppers to a large bowl and cover with plastic wrap. Let stand until cool enough to handle. (This helps to loosen the skins for easy peeling.)

In a saucepan, place the tea bags and potato in 3 cups cold water. Bring to a boil, reduce the heat and simmer until the potato is tender, about 30 minutes. Drain and let it stand until cool enough to handle. Peel the potato and cut into 1-inch cubes.

Scrape off the charred skin of the bell peppers with a knife. Core and seed each pepper. Cut peppers into 2-inch squares. Mix peppers and potato in a salad bowl. Spoon Thai Sauce over the salad and garnish with the green onion.

Makes 2 servings

Green Tea–Sautéed Vegetables

The first time I was served steamed vegetables at an American restaurant, I was shocked by what they had done to the poor vegetables. They had been steamed so long that the vegetables had been drained of life.

For a vibrant vegetable dish, try this flavorful and colorful combination of broccoli and zucchini. Don't be surprised if your children ask for seconds on the vegetables. See page 10 for ways to use the tea used to brew the liquid.

2 TABLESPOONS CANOLA OIL

2 TEASPOONS FINELY CHOPPED FRESH RED CHILE PEPPER

1 TEASPOON GRATED LEMON PEEL

1 TEASPOON LOOSE TEA LEAVES, PREFERABLY GUNPOWDER

4 CUPS BROCCOLI FLORETS

1 CUP YELLOW ZUCCHINI OR YELLOW SUMMER SQUASH, CUT INTO ¼-INCH DIAGONAL SLICES

½ CUP BREWED GREEN TEA (PAGE 7)

¼ CUP (1-INCH) RED BELL PEPPER SQUARES

SALT AND BLACK PEPPER, TO TASTE

Add the oil to a nonstick wok or cooking pan over medium-high heat and swirl the pan to coat. Add the chile pepper, lemon peel and tea leaves and stir-fry until fragrant, about 1 minute.

Add the broccoli and zucchini and stir-fry for 2 minutes. Add the tea and bell pepper and season with salt and pepper. Cook until most of the liquid evaporates, about 1 minute. Serve hot.

Makes 4 servings

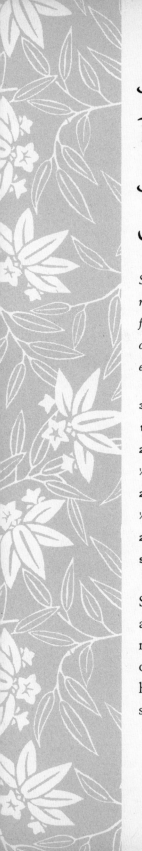

Stir-Fried Bok Choy with Shiitake Mushrooms

Shanghai or baby bok choy is sweeter and more tender than regular bok choy. I have seen it at the health food store and the farmer's market. Many restaurants cook this dish with a base of chicken broth. Vegetarians will be happy to know they can enjoy a vegetarian version of this Cantonese delicacy.

3 DRIED SHIITAKE MUSHROOMS

1 POUND BABY BOK CHOY OR REGULAR BOK CHOY

2 TABLESPOONS CANOLA OIL

½ TABLESPOON LOOSE GREEN TEA

2 CLOVES GARLIC, MINCED

½ TABLESPOON RICE WINE

2 TABLESPOONS RICE MILK OR SOYMILK

SALT AND BLACK PEPPER, TO TASTE

Soak the mushrooms in warm water until softened, about 15 minutes. Rinse the undersides of the soaked mushrooms under cold running water to clean them of any dirt or sand. Squeeze the mushrooms in your hand to thoroughly wring out the water. Discard the stems. Cut the caps into 2-inch chunks.

Wash and drain the bok choy. Cut it lengthwise into 3-inch pieces.

Heat the oil in a nonstick cooking pan or wok over medium-high heat and swirl the pan to coat. Add the tea leaves and stir-fry until fragrant, about 30 seconds. Add the garlic and mushrooms and stir-fry until fragrant, about 1 minute.

Add the bok choy, and cover immediately to prevent oil splattering. Give the pan two good shakes and cook for 30 seconds. Remove the cover and stir-fry until bok choy leaves turn green and soften. Add the rice wine and rice milk and stir-fry for 1 minute. Season with salt and pepper. Serve hot.

Makes 4 servings

Spicy Green Tea Grilled Broccoli

This is one of my favorite dishes. It is quick and easy. The green tea and chile pepper help to bring out the best flavor of the broccoli. Serve with steamed rice or noodles.

1 POUND BROCCOLI

2 TABLESPOONS CANOLA OIL

1 TABLESPOON LOOSE GREEN TEA

1 FRESH RED CHILE PEPPER, CUT INTO 2-INCH-LONG THIN STRIPS

1 TABLESPOON RICE WINE OR DRY SHERRY

SALT AND BLACK PEPPER, TO TASTE

Peel the broccoli stalks: With a paring knife, make a small cut at the bottom of the stem, grab a bit of skin between your thumb and the knife and pull away from you. The tough skin will separate easily from the stalk. Repeat around the stalk until all skin is removed. Cut the broccoli stems in half lengthwise, then into 1-inch pieces. Cut the florets in half. Wash and drain.

Heat the oil in a nonstick stovetop grill over medium heat and swirl to coat the surface. Add the green tea and grill until fragrant, about 30 seconds. Add the chile and broccoli and grill until broccoli browns, about 5 minutes. Turn occasionally with a spatula to grill all sides of the broccoli. Add the wine and season with salt and pepper. Grill for 2 more minutes. Serve hot.

Makes 4 servings

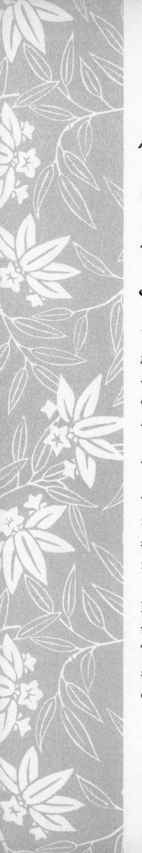

Tofu and Asparagus in Spicy Lemon-Basil Sauce

When spring comes and asparagus is in season, I like to pre-pare this dish. It is a great way to welcome this beautiful sea-son. Use the most tender asparagus and the best green tea you can find. The recipe only calls for the tips of the spears, but do save the rest for another dish.

4 BAGS GREEN TEA

1 (12-OZ.) PACKAGE REDUCED-FAT EXTRA FIRM SILKEN TOFU, CUT INTO 1-INCH SQUARES

½ CUP ½-INCH-LONG ASPARAGUS TIPS

3 FRESH CILANTRO SPRIGS, LEAVES ONLY

½ CUP SPICY LEMON-BASIL SAUCE (PAGE 47)

Bring 4 cups of water to a boil in a steamer pot. Add the tea bags. Place tofu on a heatproof bowl or plate. Top with the asparagus and cilantro leaves. Place on a steamer rack over boiling water. Cover and steam over high heat for 3 minutes.

Transfer tofu and asparagus to a serving bowl.

Pour the sauce over the asparagus and tofu and toss lightly to mix. Serve chilled.

Makes 4 to 6 servings

Green Beans with Spicy Topping

I love to cook this dish whenever I can find small and tender fresh green beans. What could be better than welcoming spring with these?

3 BAGS GREEN TEA

4 CUPS FRESH SMALL GREEN BEANS, TRIMMED

1 TABLESPOON CANOLA OIL

1 FRESH CAYENNE CHILE PEPPER, MINCED

½ CUP OYSTER MUSHROOMS, MINCED

2 GREEN ONIONS, WHITE PART ONLY, MINCED

SALT AND BLACK PEPPER, TO TASTE

1 TABLESPOON RICE VINEGAR

1 TEASPOON SESAME OIL

In a big pot, bring 4 cups water to a boil over high heat. Add the tea bags. Place a steamer rack in the pot and add beans. Steam beans until softened, about 8 minutes.

Heat the oil in a nonstick wok or cooking pan over medium heat and swirl to coat the pan. Add the chile pepper, mushrooms and onions and sauté for 1 minute. Season with salt, pepper and rice vinegar and stir-fry for 1 minute more.

Place steamed beans on a serving plate. Top with mushroom mixture. Drizzle with sesame oil and serve hot.

Makes 4 servings

Soybeans in the Pods

As a youth in China I spent many summer days snacking on sweet, delicious soybeans. I remember those summer nights under the grape trellis snacking on soybeans with my friends and wondering how ice cream tasted. Today in America I could feast on all the ice cream I want, but I still favor soybeans. They are packed with soy protein and are fun to eat. They make a great side dish or snack.

With all the information about soy's health benefits, do you ever wonder what you can do to increase soy in your diet? Start with this recipe.

4 BAGS GREEN TEA

1 POUND FRESH OR FROZEN EDAMAME (GREEN SOYBEANS IN THE PODS)

½ CUP SPICY LEMON-BASIL SAUCE (PAGE 47)

Bring 5 cups water to a boil in a large pot. Add the tea bags. Add the soybeans and bring back to a boil. Boil, uncovered, until the soybeans turn bright green, 5 to 7 minutes.

Drain soybeans and rinse under cold water to stop the cooking process. Discard tea bags.

Dip soybeans in the sauce and suck the beans into your mouth, discarding the pods. Provide bowls for the empty pods.

Makes 4 to 6 servings

Shelled Green Soybeans with Baked Tofu

This was one of the summer dishes our family ate most frequently in China. Early in the morning I would sit with my grandmother under our shady fruit tree, shelling soybeans and listening to her fascinating stories.

To shorten the preparation time, look for frozen shelled soybeans in your local health food stores or Asian markets. Serve over steamed rice or noodles. See page 10 for ways to use the tea used to brew the liquid.

5 CUPS BREWED GREEN TEA (PAGE 7)

2 CUPS SHELLED GREEN SOYBEANS

1 TABLESPOON CANOLA OIL

2 TABLESPOONS CHILE-GARLIC OIL (PAGE 45)

1 (8-OZ.) PACKAGE ORIENTAL OR OTHER FLAVORED BAKED TOFU, CUT INTO 1-INCH CUBES

3 GREEN ONIONS, WHITE PART ONLY, CUT INTO 1-INCH LENGTHS

½ CUP MINCED RED BELL PEPPER

1 TABLESPOON LOW-SODIUM SOY SAUCE

1 TEASPOON LEMON JUICE

1 TEASPOON SESAME OIL

SALT AND BLACK PEPPER, TO TASTE

Place the green tea in a big pot and bring to a boil. Add the soybeans. Boil, uncovered, until bright green, about 3 minutes. Drain.

Heat the canola oil and Chile-Garlic Oil in a nonstick cooking pan or wok over medium-high heat and swirl the pan to coat. Add the tofu and stir-fry until golden-brown, about 2 minutes.

Add the soybeans and stir-fry for 1 minute. Add the green onions, bell pepper, soy sauce, lemon juice and sesame oil. Stir-fry until heated through, 1 to 2 minutes. Season with salt and black pepper.

Make 4 servings

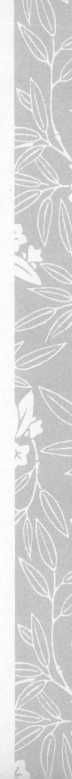

Tofu and Pineapple Kebabs

Do you know that soy is loaded with plant estrogens and may help women reduce the symptoms of menopause? Women in China and Japan consume more soy in their diet than do women in the West. In the United States about 46 percent of menopausal women try hormone-replacement therapy, while in Japan only 6 percent do.

Page 10 gives ways to use the tea used to brew the liquid.

1 (1-LB.) BLOCK EXTRA-FIRM TOFU, DRAINED

32 CHERRY TOMATOES

1 FRESH PINEAPPLE, PEELED, CORED AND CUT
INTO ¾ INCH CUBES

GREEN TEA–PINEAPPLE MARINADE

½ CUP BREWED GREEN TEA (PAGE 7)

¼ CUP PINEAPPLE JUICE CONCENTRATE

2 TABLESPOONS FRESH MINT, CHOPPED

3 CLOVES GARLIC, MINCED

1 TABLESPOON MINCED GINGER ROOT

1 TABLESPOON OLIVE OIL

SALT AND WHITE PEPPER, TO TASTE

Make the marinade: Combine all ingredients in a blender and process until pureed.

Preheat the oven to 400F (205C). Place the tofu on an oiled plate and bake for 30 minutes.

Cut the tofu into 8 equal squares: Slice in half lengthwise, then cut each piece into quarters.

Marinate the tofu and tomatoes in the marinade in the refrigerator for 2 hours, turning gently two times. Soak 8 (10-inch) bamboo skewers in water at least 30 minutes.

Preheat a stovetop or regular grill. Thread the ingredients onto skewers, alternating tofu, tomatoes and pineapple. Reserve the marinade.

Place the kebabs on the grill and cook until the tomatoes brown, 2 to 3 minutes on each side. Brush the remaining marinade on the kebabs before serving.

Make 8 servings

VARIATION

YOU CAN ALSO PLACE THE KEBABS ON A SHEET OF FOIL COATED WITH NONSTICK COOKING SPRAY. BROIL UNDER A PREHEATED BROILER, 2 TO 3 INCHES FROM THE HEAT, FOR 2 TO 3 MINUTES ON EACH SIDE.

TIP

BAKING THE TOFU HELPS STABILIZE IT. USE REGULAR TOFU, BECAUSE SILKEN TOFU WILL BE TOO FRAGILE.

Teriyaki-Ginger Baked Tofu

Use this easy recipe to make your own flavored baked tofu. You can vary the flavoring ingredients to suit your taste.

3 BAGS GREEN TEA

½ CUP TERIYAKI SAUCE

2 TABLESPOONS LEMON JUICE

1 TABLESPOON MINCED GINGER ROOT

1 (1-LB.) BLOCK EXTRA-FIRM REGULAR OR LOW-FAT FRESH TOFU

Brew the tea bags in ½ cup water for 6 minutes. Discard the tea bags. (See page 10 for ways to use the tea.)

Combine the tea, teriyaki sauce, lemon juice and ginger in a plastic container.

Place a small plate on top of the tofu and gently press out the water. Slice the tofu lengthwise in half. Add the tofu to the tea mixture. Cover and refrigerate overnight, making sure the sauce covers the tofu.

Preheat oven to 350F (175C). Drain tofu and place on a greased nonstick baking sheet. Bake the tofu for 30 minutes, or until firm and compact.

Makes about 12 ounces

Hearty Rice and Noodles

With my busy schedule, I always make extra rice and refrigerate it in a tightly covered container. It will last up to five days.

Rice

On weeknights, stir-fry some leftover rice with some precut meat, flavored tofu or frozen shrimp and a bag of salad or frozen vegetables. In minutes, you are enjoying a nutritious meal with proteins, vitamins and carbohydrates. Rice can easily be reheated in a steamer or microwave oven. Try adding a couple of bags of jasmine green tea to the steamer. You will enjoy the flavored rice.

The easiest way to cook rice is use an electric rice cooker (see page 14). If you don't have a rice cooker, the following steps will help you cook tender, fluffy rice. I have found the best pots in which to cook rice are Le Creuset's enameled cast-iron saucepans and round French ovens. The cast iron retains heat and is energy efficient, promoting even cooking at low temperatures.

Noodles

Store noodles in a tightly sealed container in a cool and dry place. One section of my pantry is devoted to dry noodles. They will keep for months. I like having lots of varieties on hand. It is like matching outfits. I select the type and size of the noodles depending on my available time and the dish I am cooking. Thin noodles for less time; rice noodles for soup; wheat noodles for stir-frying. Most of the time you can substitute different types of noodles for each other.

Dried rice noodles must be soaked in warm water until soft before cooking.

Basic Cooked Rice

Use this method if you don't have an automatic rice cooker. Let the rice cool before stir-frying. Stir-frying warm rice causes it to stick together and to the pan.

1 CUP LONG-GRAIN RICE

2 CUPS COLD WATER

Place rice and cold water in a deep saucepot.

Bring the rice and water to a boil over medium-high heat. Boil about 3 minutes, stirring occasionally.

Reduce the heat to low; partially cover the pot. Let it simmer till rice is soft and tender, 20 to 25 minutes.

Makes about 3 cups cooked rice

VARIATIONS

FOR 1 CUP SHORT-GRAIN RICE, USE 1½ CUPS COLD WATER.
FOR 1 CUP GLUTINOUS (SWEET) RICE, USE 1¼ CUPS COLD WATER.

Teriyaki Rice, Vegetables and Beef Cups

This dish was one of my childhood favorites. The flavor of plain rice combined with tea and cilantro will give you a fine long-lasting memory. Traditionally, the Chinese use bamboo cups. If you don't have them, use custard cups, small heatproof glass bowls or even teacups.

4 DRIED SHIITAKE MUSHROOMS

2 TABLESPOONS TERIYAKI SAUCE

1½ TABLESPOONS LIME JUICE

4 OUNCES BEEF EYE OF ROUND, THINLY SLICED

2 TABLESPOONS CANOLA OIL

2 TABLESPOONS PEANUTS

4 TEASPOONS GREEN TEA LEAVES

1 TABLESPOON MINCED GINGER ROOT

4 CLOVES GARLIC, MINCED

½ CUP MINCED CARROT

3 CUPS COOKED GLUTINOUS (SWEET) RICE

4 GREEN ONIONS, MINCED

2 TABLESPOONS LOW-SODIUM SOY SAUCE

SALT AND WHITE PEPPER, TO TASTE

4 BAGS GREEN TEA

3 FRESH CILANTRO SPRIGS, LEAVES ONLY

¼ CUP ROASTED PEANUTS

Soak the mushrooms in hot water until softened, about 15 minutes. Rinse the undersides of the soaked mushrooms under cold running water to clean them of any dirt or sand. Squeeze the mushrooms in your hand to thoroughly wring out the water. Discard the stems. Thinly slice the caps.

Combine the teriyaki sauce and lime juice in a bowl. Add the beef. Cover and refrigerate for 30 minutes or longer.

Preheat the broiler. Drain the beef, discarding marinade. Place beef on a piece of foil. Broil about 4 inches from the heat until browned, about 5 minutes. Let cool and chop into ½-inch squares.

Heat the oil in a nonstick wok or cooking pan over medium-high heat and swirl to coat pan. Add the peanuts, tea leaves, ginger and garlic and stir-fry until fragrant, about 2 minutes. Add the mushrooms and carrot and stir-fry for 3 minutes. Add the beef, rice, green onions and soy sauce. Mix thoroughly. Season with salt and pepper. Remove from the heat.

Grease the inside of 6 cups. Divide the rice mixture among the cups, using about ¾ cup for each, packing firmly.

In a big pot, bring 4 cups water to a boil over high heat. Place the tea bags in the water. Place the rice-filled cups on a steamer rack over the tea and steam for 10 minutes. Place a serving plate on top of each cup, turn upside down and remove cups. Garnish with cilantro leaves and roasted peanuts.

Makes 6 servings

Colorful Fried Rice

If you want to get your kids to eat healthy, try this dish. Feel free to replace the tomato with a fruit of their choice. For a spicy version, serve with Chile-Garlic Oil (page 45).

1 GREEN ONION

2 EGGS

SALT AND BLACK PEPPER, TO TASTE

3 TABLESPOONS CANOLA OIL

3 CLOVES GARLIC, CHOPPED

1 TABLESPOON LOOSE GREEN TEA

½ CUP COOKED BAY SHRIMP

1 MEDIUM TOMATO, SEEDED AND CHOPPED INTO 2-INCH CUBES

½ CUP 1-INCH PINEAPPLE CUBES

3 CUPS COOKED RICE

2 TEASPOONS SESAME OIL

Divide the white and green parts of the green onion. Mince the white part for the egg mixture. Mince the green part and set aside for the garnish.

Mix the white part of the onion with the eggs. Beat well. Season the egg mixture with salt and pepper, and mix thoroughly.

Heat 2 tablespoons of the canola oil in a nonstick wok or cooking pan over medium-high heat and swirl to coat pan. Pour in the egg mixture. Let cook until firm and brown, about 30 seconds. Turn the egg

and brown the other side. Break eggs into small pieces with the spatula. Remove and set aside.

Heat the remaining 1 tablespoon canola oil in the wok over medium-high heat. Add the garlic and tea and stir-fry until fragrant, about 1 minute. Add the shrimp and tomato and stir-fry for 1 minute. Mix in the pineapple, stir-fry for 30 seconds, then mix in the rice. Stir-fry until the rice is heated through. Season with salt and pepper. Mix in the eggs and sesame oil. Garnish with reserved green onion. Serve hot.

Makes 4 to 6 servings

TIP

IF THE OIL IS HOT ENOUGH, THE EGGS WILL BE FLUFFY. IF THE OIL IS NOT HOT ENOUGH, THEY WON'T FLUFF UP AND WON'T BE AS FLAVORFUL.

Rice Balls

When the time came for the "re-education of bourgeois children" during China's Cultural Revolution, my grandmother prepared this dish for me to take to the countryside. I always ended up sharing it with my best friends. Today, I send my son to school with this same dish. The difference is that he never wants to share. To prevent sticking, rinse hands in cold water before handling the rice. You can also serve the rice balls with one of the sauces on pages 39 to 50.

4 BAGS GREEN TEA

2 CUPS SPINACH LEAVES, LARGE STEMS REMOVED

1 TABLESPOON CANOLA OIL

1 CUP SMALL CUBES FLAVORED BAKED TOFU
(PAGE 141 OR PURCHASED)

¼ CUP MINCED CARROT

2 GREEN ONIONS (GREEN PART ONLY), MINCED

3 CUPS COOKED GLUTINOUS (SWEET) RICE

1 TABLESPOON LOW-SODIUM SOY SAUCE

1 TEASPOON WHITE PEPPER

1 TABLESPOON SESAME OIL

DASH OF SALT, TO TASTE

In a medium pot, bring 4 cups water to a boil. Add 3 of the tea bags and spinach leaves. Boil until the spinach is soft, about 30 seconds (be careful not to overcook). Drain and rinse under cold water. Squeeze out excess water and mince.

Heat the canola oil in a nonstick wok or cooking pan over medium-high heat. Add the tofu and carrot

and stir-fry until tofu is golden brown, about 2 minutes. Add the spinach and green onions and stir-fry for 1 minute. Stir in the rice, soy sauce and pepper. Tear open the remaining bag of green tea and pour the contents into the pan. Add the sesame oil. Mix thoroughly and cook until the rice heats through. Season with salt.

Place 3 to 4 tablespoons of the rice mixture in the center of a 10 x 8-inch piece of plastic wrap. Pack tightly into a ball with your hands. Repeat with the remaining rice mixture and more plastic wrap. Serve warm or cold. You can leave the plastic wrapping on until served.

Makes 8 to 10 balls (2 cups)

VARIATION

YOU CAN REPLACE THE SPINACH LEAVES WITH BOK CHOY LEAVES.

Chicken Chow Mein

I find that precut chicken for stir-frying in the markets is usually in very large pieces. Since stir-frying is fast cooking, it is best to cut the chicken into smaller pieces. The chicken will cook more evenly and pick up more of the flavors of the sauce and other ingredients. I do buy the precut chicken to save time, but I cut them smaller before cooking.

1 TEASPOON CORNSTARCH

2 TABLESPOONS SPICY LEMON-BASIL SAUCE (PAGE 47)

8 OUNCES BONELESS, SKINLESS CHICKEN BREAST,
CUT INTO 2-TO-3-INCH-LONG MATCHSTICK-SIZE
STRIPS

4 OUNCES DRIED FLAT RICE STICK NOODLES

2 TABLESPOONS CANOLA OIL

3 CLOVES GARLIC, MINCED

1 TEASPOON LOOSE GREEN TEA OR CONTENTS OF
1 BAG GREEN TEA

1 CUP FRESH SHIITAKE OR OYSTER MUSHROOMS, CUT
INTO 3-INCH-LONG MATCHSTICK-SIZE STRIPS

1 LARGE RED BELL PEPPER, CUT INTO 3-INCH-LONG
MATCHSTICK-SIZE STRIPS

6 GREEN ONIONS (WHITE PART ONLY), CUT DIAGONALLY
INTO 3-INCH-LONG MATCHSTICK-SIZE STRIPS

1 TABLESPOON FISH SAUCE

¼ CUP BREWED GREEN TEA (PAGE 7)

SALT AND BLACK PEPPER, TO TASTE

FRESH CILANTRO LEAVES

Dissolve the cornstarch in the sauce. Add the chicken and toss to combine. Cover and refrigerate for 30 minutes. Drain and set aside.

Soak the noodles in the hot water until soft, 15 to 20 minutes. Drain and set aside.

Arrange all ingredients near the cooking area. Heat the oil in a nonstick wok or cooking pan over medium-high heat and swirl to coat pan. Add the garlic, tea leaves and mushrooms and stir-fry until fragrant, about 1 minute.

Add the chicken and stir-fry until chicken is no longer pink, about 2 minutes. Add the bell pepper and green onions and stir-fry for 30 seconds. Mix in the noodles, fish sauce and brewed tea. Season with salt and pepper. Cook, stirring occasionally, until noodles are heated through. Garnish with cilantro leaves.

Makes 4 to 6 servings

Spicy Thai Shrimp Noodles

No more midnight craving for Thai food! Now you can make your own at home. Feel free to substitute tofu, chicken or mussels for the shrimp.

1 (9-OZ.) PACKAGE FRESH FETTUCCINE

2 TABLESPOONS CANOLA OIL

2 TEASPOONS LOOSE GREEN TEA

8 OUNCES RAW MEDIUM SHRIMP, SHELLED AND DEVEINED

3 GREEN ONIONS (GREEN AND WHITE PARTS), CUT INTO
2-INCH LENGTHS

½ CUP RED BELL PEPPER, CUT INTO 2-INCH-LONG
MATCHSTICK-SIZE STRIPS

½ CUP YELLOW BELL PEPPER, CUT INTO 2-INCH-LONG
MATCHSTICK-SIZE STRIPS

⅓ CUP SPICY CILANTRO SAUCE (PAGE 44)

1 TABLESPOON FISH SAUCE

2 TABLESPOONS MINCED FRESH CILANTRO

SALT AND BLACK PEPPER, TO TASTE

3 TABLESPOONS ROASTED PEANUTS, MINCED

Cook the noodles according to the package instructions. Drain and rinse under cold water to stop the cooking process and prevent sticking.

Heat the oil in a nonstick wok or pan over medium-high heat and swirl to coat pan. Add the tea leaves and fry until fragrant, about 30 seconds. Add the shrimp and stir-fry until shrimp are pink, about

1 minute. Add the green onions and bell peppers and stir-fry for another minute.

Stir in the noodles and stir-fry for 30 seconds. Add the Spicy Cilantro Sauce and fish sauce. Stir-fry until the noodles are heated through, about 2 minutes. Stir in the cilantro and season with salt and white pepper. Serve hot or cold, garnished with peanuts.

Makes 4 serving

Cold Noodles in Peanut Sauce

This dish makes a great lunch and summer picnic. You can make the sauce and cook the noodles ahead of time, then put the dish together at the last minute.

6 BAGS GREEN TEA

8 OUNCES FRESH OR DRIED LINGUINE

1 TABLESPOON CANOLA OIL

4 OUNCES FLAVORED BAKED TOFU (PAGE 141 OR PUCHASED), CUT INTO SMALL CUBES

1 CUP THINLY SLICED CABBAGE

1 SMALL LEEK, WHITE PART ONLY, CUT INTO LONG MATCHSTICK-SIZE STRIPS

1 SMALL RED BELL PEPPER, CUT INTO LONG MATCHSTICK-SIZE PIECES

1 LARGE MILD GREEN CHILE, CUT INTO LONG MATCHSTICK-SIZE PIECES

½ CUP CURRY PEANUT SAUCE (PAGE 48)

SALT AND BLACK PEPPER, TO TASTE

4 FRESH CILANTRO SPRIGS, CUT INTO 1-INCH-LONG PIECES

In a large pot, bring 6 cups water to a boil. Turn off the heat and add the tea bags. Let brew for 2 minutes. Discard the tea bags. (See page 10 for ways to use the tea in the bags.)

Bring the tea to a boil. Add the noodles and cook according to the package directions. Drain and rinse under cold water.

Heat the oil in a nonstick wok or cooking pan over medium-high heat and swirl to coat the pan. Add the tofu and stir-fry until golden brown, 1 to 2 minutes. Add the cabbage, leek, bell pepper and chile and stir-fry until cabbage softens, 1 to 2 minutes. Add the noodles and sauce and mix thoroughly. Season with salt and pepper. Serve cold, garnished with cilantro.

Makes 4 servings

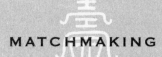

MATCHMAKING

In the old days, many Chinese marriages were arranged by matchmakers. The matchmakers found a suitable family and set up the first meeting for the young couple and their families. Tea was always served by the prospective bride. At the meeting the mother of the prospective groom examined the young woman closely. If she drank the tea before the leaves sank to the bottom, she was considered impatient. The marriage very likely would not occur between the young couple. If instead she could wait until the hot water unfurled the tea leaves and they sank to the bottom of the teacup, she would be approved for her good manners.

Luckily, my American mother-in-law served me tea made with tea bags the first time we met.

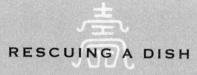

RESCUING A DISH

Choose only one option if more than one is given.

TOO BLAND:

+ For vegetables—add a dash of salt, hot chile pepper oil or chicken broth.
+ For meats—add a dash of soy sauce and vinegar or minced garlic.
+ For seafood—add a dash of fish sauce, rice wine or minced ginger.

TOO SALTY:

+ Add more fresh or frozen vegetables to the dish.
+ Add a diced peeled potato. It will absorb the excess salt.
+ Add a dash of vinegar or sugar.

TOO MUCH OIL:

+ Add more fresh vegetables.
+ Drain off the excess oil.

TOO LITTLE OIL:

+ Use the spatula to push the food to the sides, create a hole in the center of the wok or cooking pan and add more oil.

STICKING TO THE PAN:

+ USE THE METHODS FOR TOO LITTLE OIL.

+ TURN DOWN THE HEAT AND ADD SOME WATER.

UNDERCOOKED:

+ RETURN FOOD TO THE PAN. COOK OVER LOW HEAT, ADDING MORE SAUCE OR WATER, IF NEEDED.

OVERCOOKED:

+ STIR IN SOME COLORFUL, EASY-TO-COOK VEGETABLES SUCH AS PEAS, MINCED BELL PEPPERS OR LEAFY VEGETABLES.

SAUCE TOO THICK:

+ REDUCE THE HEAT TO LOW. STIR IN A LITTLE WATER WHILE THE SAUCE IS STILL SIMMERING. ADD WATER, 2 TABLE-SPOONS AT A TIME, AS NEEDED.

SAUCE TOO THIN:

+ REDUCE THE HEAT TO MEDIUM-LOW. DISSOLVE 1 TEASPOON CORNSTARCH IN 1 TABLESPOON COLD WATER AND STIR INTO THE SAUCE. COOK, STIRRING, UNTIL THE SAUCE BEGINS TO THICKEN. REPEAT THIS PROCEDURE AS NECESSARY.

NOT ATTRACTIVE:

+ USE COLORFUL FRUITS AND VEGETABLES AS GARNISH. BE IMAGINATIVE! A BEAUTIFUL SERVING DISH IS ALWAYS A BIG PLUS.

Delectable Desserts and Beverages

What food are you craving? This question came up in a gathering of friends. Chocolate, cheesecake, spicy Thai food?

My craving is Sweet Eight-Treasure Rice Pudding. Food is often associated with important memories and events in our lives. During many years of my childhood, food was strictly rationed. The only time we could eat this treat was at the Chinese New Year. I remember many times when I wished that I could eat this dish whenever I wanted. Now when I crave sweets, about once or twice a month, I cook this dish.

Desserts

Need an easy dessert? A friend who took a cooking class from a sushi chef told me this secret to making an easy green tea ice cream. Soften 1 cup vanilla ice cream and stir in ½ teaspoon matcha tea (green tea powder used for the Japanese tea ceremony); then put the ice cream back in the freezer. Once it's firm, it's ready to serve. Easy—but you can let your friends think you made it from scratch!

Beverages

Next time you want something sweet, reach for a sweet drink rather than a dessert, and try one of the fruit and green tea drinks. My favorite is the Green Tea, Mango and Yogurt Smoothie. These drinks are low in fat and sugar yet full of flavor, with a healthy hint of flavored green tea.

Cooking is an art. Think of it as painting a masterpiece, using the many fruit- or jasmine-flavored green teas plus some of your favorite ingredients to create your own edible creations.

Green Tea Ice Cream

Another example of how "bland" tofu can be more than just a health-conscious foodstuff. The kiwi fruit adds a touch of green to the ice cream, but feel free to substitute other fruit. Being a vegetarian doesn't mean you have to bypass this treat. Traditionally, ice cream requires cow's milk and cream. I have experimented a bit and found that with soymilk and soy whipped topping, it comes out just as delicious.

1 CUP PLAIN OR VANILLA SOYMILK

4 BAGS FRUIT-FLAVORED GREEN TEA

1 (12-OZ.) PACKAGE LOW-FAT FIRM SILKEN TOFU

½ CUP CREAMED HAZELNUT HONEY OR REGULAR HONEY

1 TABLESPOON VANILLA EXTRACT

2 KIWI FRUIT, PEELED AND DICED INTO CHUNKS

1 CUP NONDAIRY WHIPPED TOPPING

2 OR 3 DROPS GREEN FOOD COLORING (OPTIONAL)

Bring the soymilk and teabags to a boil in a medium saucepan. Reduce heat and simmer for 5 minutes. Stir frequently to prevent scorching. Remove from heat and let cool. Use two spoons to gently squeeze absorbed milk out of tea bags and discard bags.

In a blender, combine the tofu, soymilk mixture, honey, vanilla, and kiwi fruit. Blend until mixture is smooth, 2 to 3 minutes.

Pour blended mixture into a bowl suitable for freezing. Gently fold the whipped topping, mixed with food coloring, if using, into the blended mixture. Cover and freeze 5 to 6 hours or until firm.

Makes 4 to 6 servings

TIP

AN EASY WAY TO MEASURE OUT THE HONEY IS TO FIRST TRANSFER THE GREEN TEA–MILK INTO A LARGE LIQUID MEASURING CUP. ADD HONEY UNTIL THE VOLUME HAS INCREASED BY ½ CUP. THE MILK WILL HELP KEEP THE HONEY FROM STICKING TO THE MEASURING CUP AS YOU POUR IT INTO THE BLENDER.

Sweet Jasmine Tea Cake

The last time I prepared this gooey-textured cake for a dinner party, half of it was gone before my guests arrived the following day. I ended up having to make one more dessert. It is my Asian friends' favorite dessert.

1½ CUPS GLUTINOUS RICE FLOUR

1 CUP REGULAR RICE FLOUR

1 CUP SUGAR

1 CUP BREWED JASMINE GREEN TEA (PAGE 7) MADE WITH 2 TEA BAGS

½ CUP MARGARINE, MELTED

CONTENTS OF 3 BAGS JASMINE GREEN TEA

In a large mixing bowl, mix the flours, sugar and brewed tea (see page 10 for ways of using the tea in the bags) until smooth. Fold in the margarine and dry tea and mix to form a smooth batter.

Coat a 10-inch-round nonstick cake pan with nonstick cooking spray. Pour in the batter.

Place the cake pan on a steamer basket. Steam over boiling water until the cake is translucent, about 25 minutes. Let the cake cool. Cut into wedges and serve.

Makes 10 servings

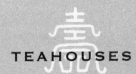

TEAHOUSES

CHINESE TEAHOUSES HAVE EXISTED AS LONG AS THERE HAS BEEN TEA. IN ANCIENT TIMES, THE OFFICERS OF THE EMPEROR'S COURT AND SCHOLARS HAD SPECIAL ROOMS FOR TEA SESSIONS. THIS ROOM WAS GENERALLY SURROUNDED BY A LOTUS POND OR LAKE, A SMALL BRIDGE, SHAPED ROCKS, TREES AND FLOWERS. TEAROOMS WERE USED FOR PLAYING CHESS, READING POETRY, PLAYING MUSIC, MEDITATION AND WATCHING NATURE.

PUBLIC TEAHOUSES EMERGED ACROSS CHINA WHEN TEA SPREAD TO THE COMMON PEOPLE. FROM MORNING TO NIGHT, PEOPLE STILL GO TO TEAHOUSES TO SAMPLE VARIOUS TEAS, RELAX, MEET FRIENDS, ENJOY TEA SNACKS OR DIM SUM, TALK BUSINESS, ARRANGE MARRIAGES AND SETTLE DISPUTES.

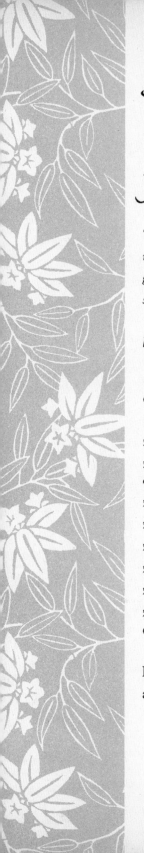

Sweet Eight-Treasure Rice Pudding

This is a popular Chinese dessert. Feel free to add more fruit; use whatever fresh fruit is in season. If you have a hard time getting your children to eat healthy desserts, this will be a good start.

See page 10 for ways of using the tea used for brewing the liquid.

1¼ CUPS BREWED FRUIT-FLAVORED GREEN TEA (PAGE 7)

1 CUP GLUTINOUS (SWEET) RICE

½ CUP CHOPPED FRESH MANGO

¼ CUP GREEN CANDIED CHERRIES, HALVED OR QUARTERED

¼ CUP RAISINS

¼ CUP DRIED TART CHERRIES

¼ CUP CHOPPED CANDIED PINEAPPLE

½ CUP CREAMY ALMOND BUTTER

¼ CUP MAPLE SYRUP

½ CUP GREEN TEA, MANGO AND YOGURT SMOOTHIE (PAGE 177; OPTIONAL)

Place the green tea and rice in a rice cooker. Cook and set aside.

Line the bottom of a 6-to-8-inch-deep bowl with

plastic wrap. Artistically arrange the mango and the other fruit on the bottom of the bowl.

Pack half of the warm rice into the bowl in an even layer, following the curve of the bowl. Spread the almond butter and maple syrup on the rice.

Pack the remaining rice over the almond butter-syrup layer. Firmly flatten the top of the rice.

Place a platter on top of the bowl and invert, holding them together. Carefully lift off the bowl and remove the plastic wrap to reveal your fruit arrangement. Spoon the smoothie on top, if using. Serve warm.

Makes 4 servings

Jasmine Almond Cookies

Enjoy these tasty delicate cookies with a cup of green tea or a scoop of your favorite frozen yogurt or ice cream. They're festive enough for any special occasion.

¼ CUP PLUS 2 TABLESPOONS REDUCED-FAT BUTTER
OR MARGARINE

¼ CUP CREAMY ALMOND BUTTER

½ CUP PLUS 2 TABLESPOONS SUGAR

1 EGG, LIGHTLY BEATEN

1 TEASPOON PURE VANILLA EXTRACT

¾ CUP ALL-PURPOSE FLOUR

CONTENTS OF 3 BAGS JASMINE GREEN TEA BAGS

½ TEASPOON BAKING SODA

⅛ TEASPOON SALT

40 UNBLANCHED WHOLE ALMONDS

Preheat oven to 350F (175C). In a large bowl, place the butter, almond butter, and sugar. Place in the oven for 3 to 5 minutes, until butter starts to soften. Beat until light and fluffy. Beat in the egg and vanilla until smooth.

Add the flour, tea, baking soda and salt to the egg mixture and beat until combined.

Spray a ½ tablespoon measuring spoon with non-stick cooking spray. Spoon balls of dough onto lightly sprayed baking sheets, about 2 inches apart. Press an almond into the center of each ball.

Bake 12 to 14 minutes or until cookies are lightly browned. Let cookies cool completely on baking sheets. Store in an airtight container.

Makes 40 cookies

TIPS

PLACING THE BUTTER, ALMOND BUTTER AND SUGAR INTO THE HOT OVEN HELPS SOFTEN THE BUTTER AND MAKES IT EASIER TO MIX.

SPRAYING THE TABLESPOON PREVENTS THE DOUGH FROM STICKING TO IT.

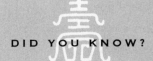

DID YOU KNOW?

FORTUNE COOKIES WERE FIRST SERVED IN 1916, THE CREATION OF A LOS ANGELES CHINESE RESTAURANT.

Melon Basket

You will have more fruit than will fit back into the melon basket. Cover and refrigerate the remaining fruit separately.

1 MEDIUM WATERMELON

1 CUP BLUEBERRIES

½ CANTALOUPE

½ CUP SEEDLESS GREEN GRAPES

½ CUP SEEDLESS RED GRAPES

1 MANGO, CUT INTO 2-INCH CHUNKS

S A U C E

½ CUP BREWED JASMINE GREEN TEA (PAGE 7)

½ CUP PINEAPPLE-COCONUT JUICE

2 TABLESPOONS MAPLE SYRUP

To make the sauce: Combine all the ingredients in a bowl. Mix well and set aside.

Cut the top portion of the watermelon to form a basket with a handle, or cut off the top and serrate the edge of the melon. Using a tablespoon or melon baller, scoop out watermelon into tablespoon-size balls.

Mix the watermelon balls and remaining fruit in a large bowl. Pour the sauce over the fruit. Spoon fruit into the melon basket. Cover and refrigerate until chilled. Serve cold.

Makes 6 to 8 servings

Three-Berry Shake

For the best color and flavor, serve immediately. It can be covered and refrigerated for one day.

½ CUP FRESH STRAWBERRIES

½ CUP FRESH BLUEBERRIES

¼ CUP FRESH RASPBERRIES

6 FROZEN FRUIT-FLAVORED GREEN TEA CUBES

2 FRESH MINT LEAVES

Place the berries and tea cubes in a blender. Blend at high speed until smooth. Pour into a glass and garnish with the mint leaves.

Makes about 1¼ cups

Peach Smoothie

For the best consistency, serve immediately. Any leftovers can be covered and frozen.

1 CUP FROZEN PEACH SLICES

½ CUP FROZEN PINEAPPLE CHUNKS

½ CUP FRUIT-FLAVORED BREWED GREEN TEA (PAGE 7)

1 ¼ TABLESPOONS HONEY

2 FRESH CHERRIES (OPTIONAL)

Place the frozen fruit, tea and honey in a blender. Blend at high speed until smooth. Pour into 2 glasses and top with the cherries, if using.

Makes 1 ½ cups

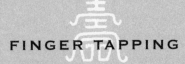

FINGER TAPPING

HAVE YOU EVER NOTICED YOUR CHINESE FRIENDS TAP THREE FINGERS ON THE TABLE WHEN YOU FILL THEIR TEACUPS? HERE IS THE STORY BEHIND IT.

THE EMPEROR OF THE QING DYNASTY LOVED TO TRAVEL AROUND THE COUNTRY ON INCOGNITO VISITS. ONE DAY HE AND HIS SERVANTS WENT INTO A TEAHOUSE IN SOUTH CHINA. IN ORDER TO PRESERVE HIS SECRET, HE TOO TOOK TURNS AT POURING TEA. HIS SURPRISED SERVANTS WANTED TO KOW-TOW (BOW) TO THEIR EMPEROR FOR THE GREAT HONOR HE GAVE TO THEM. THE EMPEROR TOLD THE SERVANTS THAT THEY COULD TAP THREE FINGERS ON THE TABLE TO EXPRESS THEIR GRATITUDE. ONE FINGER REPRESENTED THEIR BOWED HEADS AND THE OTHER TWO REPRESENTED THEIR PROS-TRATED ARMS.

AFTER THAT THE CHINESE PEOPLE ADOPTED FINGER TAP-PING AS A WAY TO EXPRESS THEIR SILENT GRATITUDE FOR TEA SERVICE. FINGER TAPPING EXPRESSES THANKS WITHOUT INTERRUPTING THE ONGOING CONVERSATIONS.

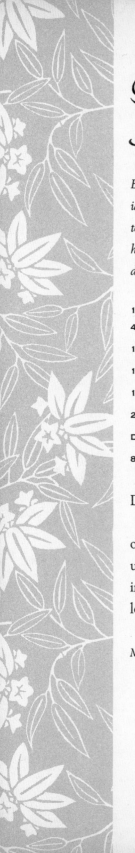

Green Tea-Soy Shake

Because both green tea and soy contain high amounts of antioxidants, I call this drink my antioxidant boost. If you have been to Boulder or another health-conscious city, chances are you have seen someone drink something like this. It makes a great dessert after a light meal, or a refreshing treat any time of day.

1 CUP FRUIT-FLAVORED GREEN TEA, BREWED WITH
4 TEA BAGS

12 FROZEN SOY CUBES (SEE TIP)

1 CUP VANILLA SOYMILK

1 CUP COCONUT-PINEAPPLE OR PINEAPPLE JUICE

2 TABLESPOONS HONEY

DASH OF CINNAMON

8 MINT LEAVES

Discard the tea bags and let the tea cool.

Blend the soy cubes at medium speed for 10 seconds. Add the soymilk, juice and honey and blend until smooth and creamy, about 15 seconds. Pour into 4 glasses and garnish with cinnamon and mint leaves.

Makes 4 cups

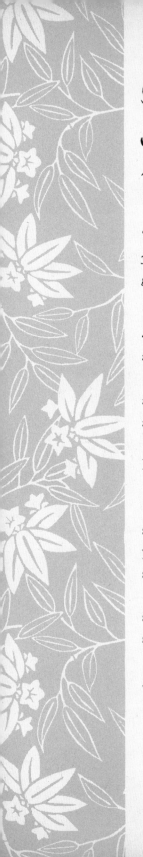

Green Tea, Mango and Yogurt Smoothie

This luxurious smoothie is my favorite. It is a great way to start your day. The green tea wakes you up gently and the protein gives you lasting energy.

1 CUP FRUIT-FLAVORED GREEN TEA, BREWED WITH 4 TEA BAGS

2 LARGE MANGOES

12 ICE CUBES

2 (6-OZ.) CARTONS APRICOT AND MANGO SOY YOGURT

2 TABLESPOONS HONEY

Discard the tea bags and let the tea cool.

Peel, seed, and cube the mangoes.

Blend the ice cubes in a blender at medium speed for 10 seconds. Add the mangoes, green tea, yogurt and honey. Blend at medium speed until smooth and frosty, about 15 seconds.

Serve immediately for best color and taste, or store in a tightly sealed container in refrigerator until serving time.

Makes 4 cups

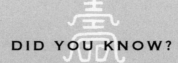

DID YOU KNOW?

ICED TEA WAS INVENTED AT THE 1904 WORLD'S FAIR IN ST. LOUIS BY A MERCHANT WHO COULDN'T SELL HIS HOT TEA IN THE SUMMER WEATHER. IN DESPERATION, HE SERVED HIS TEA WITH ICE. THIRSTY CROWDS FLOCKED AROUND HIS STAND, AND SINCE THEN AMERICANS HAVE BEEN DRINKING ICED TEA.

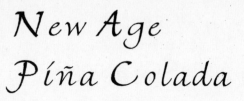

New Age
Piña Colada

This is the second piña colada recipe I created. One summer evening, I served my first "generation" to my husband, Greg, and neighbors Dan and Valerie. Greg suggested adding tofu, and Dan suggested adding more ice. Valerie voted for this creation. By the time we finished experimenting, we all felt chilled.

1 CUP FRUIT-FLAVORED GREEN TEA, BREWED WITH
4 TEA BAGS

1 CUP FROZEN PINEAPPLE JUICE CUBES

1 CUP ICE CUBES

1 CUP COCONUT-PINEAPPLE JUICE

½ (12-OZ.) PACKAGE SOFT SILKEN TOFU

3 TABLESPOONS HONEY

Discard the tea bags (see page 10 for ways to use the tea in the bags) and let the tea cool.

Blend pineapple cubes and ice in a blender until ice is crushed.

Add the tea, juice, tofu and honey. Blend on high speed until smooth and frosty, about 2 minutes. Serve immediately for the best color and taste.

Makes 3 cups

Watermelon-Banana Smoothie

Next time you are about to reach for a soft drink, how about trying this unusually delicious drink? While satisfying your thirst, you will also get important nutrients.

1 CUP FRUIT-FLAVORED GREEN TEA, BREWED WITH
4 TEA BAGS

8 FROZEN VANILLA SOYMILK CUBES (SEE TIP, PAGE 176)

2 CUPS CUBED SEEDLESS WATERMELON

2 FROZEN BANANAS, SLICED

1 TABLESPOON HONEY

Discard the tea bags and let the tea cool.

Blend the frozen soy cubes in a blender at medium speed until crushed, about 10 seconds. Add the remaining ingredients, and blend at high speed until smooth and frothy, about 15 seconds.

Pour into glasses and serve immediately for best color and taste.

Makes 3 ½ cups

Resources

In researching this book I tested many products. I found those made by the following companies to be superior. I've listed the companies' phone numbers and Web sites and/or mailing addresses for your convenience.

Teas and Teapots

Celestial Seasonings
4600 Sleepytime Drive
Boulder, CO 80301-3292
800-525-0347
www.celestialseasonings.com
Bagged green teas, Yixing teapots

Lipton Tea
Lipton Products by Mail
P.O. Box 3000
Grand Rapids, MN 55745-3000
800-697-7887
www.liptont.com
Bagged green tea

R. C. Bigelow
210 Black Rock Turnpike
Fairfield, CT 06432
888-244-3569
www.bigelowtea.com
Bagged and loose green tea

The Republic of Tea
8 Digital Drive, Suite 100
Novato, CA 94949
888-T-LEAVES
www.therepublicoftea.com
Bagged and loose green tea

Salada Green Tea
REDCO, Inc.
P.O. Box 1027
Little Falls, NY 13365
800-645-1190
www.greentea.com
Bagged green tea

Starbucks
800-STARBUC
www.starbucks.com
Loose and bagged green tea

Water and Leaves Company
690 Broadway Street
Redwood City, CA 94063-9512
800-699-4753
www.wayoftea.com
Loose tea, Yixing teapots

Yixing.com Teapots
117 E. Louisa Street, Suite 286
Seattle, WA 98102
206-320-1389
206-374-2104 Fax
www.yixing.com
Teapots

Miscellaneous Organic Foods

Eden Foods, Inc.
701 Tecumseh Road
Clinton, MI 49236
800-248-0320
www.eden-foods.com
Bottled sauces and other foods

Cookware

Calphalon Corporation
P.O. Box 583
Toledo, OH 43697-0583
800-809-7267
www.calphalon.com
Nonstick chef's pan with cover,
wok, round grill pan, 3½-quart
saucepan with cover

Le Creuset of America, Inc.
P.O. Box 67
Early Branch, SC 29916
800-827-1789
www.lecreuset.com
Teakettles, spatulas, saucepans

Scanpan USA Inc.
10 Industrial Avenue
Mahwah, NJ 07430
201-818-2280
www.scanpan.com
Stack N Steam steamer

Zojirushi American Corporation
6259 Bandini Boulevard
Commerce, CA 90040-3113
800-733-6270
www.zojirushi.com
Rice cooker

Tofu

Mori-Nu
Morinaga Nutritional Foods, Inc.
2050 West 190th Street,
   Suite 110
Torrance, CA 90504
800-699-8638
www.morinu.com/welcome.html
Silken tofu (soft, firm, extra-firm)

White Wave
1990 N. 57th Court
Boulder, CO 80301
www.whitewave.com
Baked tofu (Italian, Mexican,
   Oriental, Thai, Snack 'n
Savory)

Kitchen Knives

Zwilling J. A. Henckels, Inc.
171 Saw Mill River Road
Hawthorne, New York
   10532-1529
www.j-a-henckels.com
Twinstar Plus Knives

Conversion Tables

Comparison to Metric Measure

When You Know	Symbol	Multiply By	To Find	Symbol
teaspoons	tsp.	5.0	milliliters	ml
tablespoons	tbsp.	15.0	milliliters	ml
fluid ounces	fl. oz.	30.0	milliliters	ml
cups	c	0.24	liters	l
pints	pt.	0.47	liters	l
quarts	qt.	0.95	liters	l
ounces	oz.	28.0	grams	g
pounds	lb.	0.45	kilograms	kg
Fahrenheit	F	5/9 (after subtracting 32)	Celsius	C

Liquid Measure to Milliliters

¼	teaspoon	=	1.25	milliliters
½	teaspoon	=	2.5	milliliters
¾	teaspoon	=	3.75	milliliters
1	teaspoon	=	5.0	milliliters
1¼	teaspoons	=	6.25	milliliters
1½	teaspoons	=	7.5	milliliters
1¾	teaspoons	=	8.75	milliliters
2	teaspoons	=	10.0	milliliters
1	tablespoon	=	15.0	milliliters
2	tablespoons	=	30.0	milliliters

Fahrenheit to Celsius

F	C
200–205	95
220–225	105
245–250	120
275	135
300–305	150
325–330	165
345–350	175
370–375	190
400–405	205
425–430	220
445–450	230
470–475	245
500	260

Liquid Measure to Liters

¼	cup	=	0.06	liters
½	cup	=	0.12	liters
¾	cup	=	0.18	liters
1	cup	=	0.24	liters
1¼	cups	=	0.3	liters
1½	cups	=	0.36	liters
2	cups	=	0.48	liters
2½	cups	=	0.6	liters
3	cups	=	0.72	liters
3½	cups	=	0.84	liters
4	cups	=	0.96	liters
4½	cups	=	1.08	liters
5	cups	=	1.2	liters
5½	cups	=	1.32	liters

Index

ABOUT THE AUTHOR

YING CHANG COMPESTINE was born in
Wuhan, a city in the People's Republic of China.
After earning a degree in English literature, she
taught English and worked as a translator. In 1990,
after relocating to the United States, Ying earned a
master's degree in sociology from the University of
Colorado.

By blending her long-time passion for Chinese
cooking and her interest in health, Ying turned her
talents toward recipe development. Ying teaches
classes in healthy cooking at the Boulder Heart
Institute in Colorado and various cooking schools
throughout the country. She has been featured on
numerous television and radio programs, and in
magazines and newspapers around the country. Feature stories have appeared in *Cooking Light* and
Woman's World magazines as well as major newspapers such as *Investor's Business Daily*, *The Atlanta
Journal-Constitution*, *The Denver Post* and the *Rocky
Mountain News*.

Additionally, Ying has been featured on
Bloomberg Radio's "Food and Wine with Peter
Elliot," and on TV's Food Network and the Discov-
ery Channel. A regular contributor to such notable
magazines as *Cooking Light*, *Self* and *Men's Health*,

she also worked as a contributing editor with a monthly food column for *healthshop.com*.

Other books by Ying include *Secrets of Fat-Free Chinese Cooking* and two books for children, *The Runaway Rice Cake* and *The Story of Chopsticks*. She lives in Boulder, Colorado, with her husband and son.